CYSTS

CAUSES, DIAGNOSIS AND TREATMENT OPTIONS

PHYSIOLOGY - LABORATORY AND CLINICAL RESEARCH

CYSTS

CAUSES, DIAGNOSIS AND TREATMENT OPTIONS

ARTURO MENDES ORTIZ
AND
AUGUSTO JIMENEZ MORENO

EDITORS

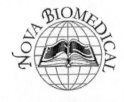

Nova Science Publishers, Inc.
New York

NOTICE TO THE READER

Library of Congress Cataloging-in-Publication Data

Library of Congress Control Number: 2012933660
ISBN: 978-1-62081-315-7

Published by Nova Science Publishers, Inc. † New York

CONTENTS

PREFACE

Cysts are pathological cavities that may or may not be lined by the epithelium and are filled with either gas, fluid or semi-solid materials. Once formed, a cyst could go away on its own or may have to be removed through surgery. In this book, the authors present current research in the study of the causes, diagnosis and treatment options of cysts. Topics discussed include recent advances in the diagnostic imaging of cysts and pseudocysts in the oral and maxillofacial region; inflammatory odontogenic cysts; cystic renal pathology; non-parasitic benign liver cysts; and the malignant potential of epidermal and verrucous cutaneous cysts.

Chapter 1 - It is sometimes difficult to differentiate cysts and pseudocysts from tumors in the jawbone on the basis of conventional radiographs. Moreover, cysts and pseudocysts that arise in soft tissue can not be detected on radiographic images without the use of contrast agents. Therefore, additional information is sometimes required to diagnose these lesions. Computed tomography and magnetic resonance imaging (CT; MRI) have been demonstrated to be very useful for depicting normal structures and pathological processes in the oral and maxillofacial region. Whereas CT is best for depicting bone structures, MRI is superior to CT at evaluating soft tissue. The contents of bone lesions might also be better visualized on MRI.

In this chapter, among the variety of lesions that occur in the oral and maxillofacial region, the authors would like to focus on those arising in the jaw or adjacent soft tissue. They present their representative CT and MRI findings and discuss the imaging characteristics that most contribute to their differential diagnosis.

1. Cysts and pseudocysts that affect the jaw
   1-a True cysts
   1-a-1) Radicular cyst
   1-a-2) Dentigerous cyst
   1-a-3) Nasopalatine duct cyst
   1-a-4) Postoperative maxillary cyst
   1-b Pseudocysts
   1-b-1) Simple bone cyst
   1-b-2) Aneurysmal bone cyst
   1-b-3) Static bone cavity
2. Cysts that affect soft tissue
   2-1) Nasolabial cyst
   2-2) Mucous retention cyst

2-3) Dermoid/epidermoid cyst

2-4) Epidermal cyst

2-5) Branchial cleft cyst

2-6) Thyroglossal duct cyst

2-7) Ranula

3. Others

3-1) Keratocystic odontogenic tumor

Chapter 2 - A radicular cyst is a pathologic cavity partially or completely lined by epithelium in an area of apical periodontitis. It is caused by infection of the root canal system, which results in an immuno-inflammatory response of the periapical tissues. A radicular cyst is presumably formed by inflammatory proliferation of epithelial cell rests in an area of apical periodontitis. Radicular cysts can be categorized into pocket and true cysts. Clinically, it is not possible to make a definitive diagnosis of a radicular cyst. The final conclusive diagnosis of a radicular cyst can only be made through histological examination of biopsy specimens. Radicular cysts [pocket and true] are of inflammatory origin and are not developmental or neoplastic. As in other infectious diseases, they should be able to regress after elimination of infection, possibly by the mechanism of apoptosis or programmed cell death. Since radicular cysts cannot be diagnosed clinically, all cyst-like inflammatory periapical lesions should be treated initially by conservative procedures, such as non-surgical root canal therapy or a decompression technique. If large cyst-like periapical lesions are treated surgically, recurrence will not occur even if the epithelial lining is not completely enucleated. Failure of radicular cysts to regress after non-surgical or surgical treatment is due to persistent intraradicular infection or reinfection of involved teeth and not due to a self-sustaining nature of the cysts.

Chapter 3 - The term "renal cyst" is rather non-specific because multiple entities can be subsumed within such categorization, with the same designating any cavity lined by epithelium. Will be "pseudocysts" those lesions formed by a cavity that lack of epithelial lining. In the case of a term so generic, it is difficult to calculate the actual incidence of renal cysts; however, the authors anticipate that this is a very frequent disease (about 5-15% of the population).

Chapter 4 - Cystic lesions of the liver represent a heterogeneous group of disorders, which differ in etiology, prevalence, and clinical manifestations.

The term liver cyst usually refers to solitary nonparasitic cysts, also known as simple cysts. However, several other cystic lesions must be distinguished from true simple cysts. Cystic lesions of the liver include simple cysts, multiple cysts arising in the setting of polycystic liver disease (PCLD), parasitic or hydatid (echinococcal) cysts, cystic tumors, and abscesses (1-3).

Chapter 5 - Liver cysts are a heterogeneous group of diseases with different aetiology and incidence. Frequently, they are asymptomatic but symptomatic cases cause similar clinical signs and symptoms. The diagnosis of these cysts is now more frequent due to the increasing number or abdominal radiological explorations (abdominal ultrasound or CT) performed for other medical reasons. They are classified as congenital, traumatic, parasitic, or neoplastic cysts. The congenital cystic tumours are the most frequent type including simple liver cyst and polycystic hepatic disease. Other less common lesions are: hepatic cystadenoma, ciliated embryonic cyst, Caroli Disease and a miscellaneous group. Liver hydatidosis is the most frequent parasitic liver cyst in many countries. The authors perform in this chapter a review of non-parasitic liver cyst focusing in most adequate treatment that includes from clinical follow-up to liver transplantation. The possibility of performing some surgical procedures by laparoscopy approach has opened some controversies in the management of liver cysts that are not well answered in medical literature.

Chapter 6 - Cysts of the oral cavity are relatively a common lesion which the oral surgeon and general dentist will have to manage during their practice. Head and neck cysts are generally a benign lesion with history of slow growth and may be asymptomatic except when they increase in size and also become secondarily infected. However, some odontogenic cyst have been reported to be aggressive especially the parakeratinized type of odontogenic keratocyst. This is one of the reasons why it was recently classified as a tumor. Also more sinister conditions like ameloblastoma, squamous cell and mucoepidermoid carcinoma have been reported to arise from the wall of a cyst. The authors' experience has shown that most of the initial histological diagnoses of cysts obtained from small tissues taken during incision biopsies are not very dependable and misleading to the surgeons as some of these lesions eventually turn out to be unicystic ameloblastoma after histological processing of post-operative specimens. Cyst linings must always be sent for histopathological examination after surgery.

It is therefore important that a dentist have a good knowledge of these important conditions so as to be able to make an accurate diagnosis and then institute an appropriate referral.

Chapter 7 - The malignant potential of cutaneous cysts is studied. The authors have examined 7 squamous cell carcinoma (SCC) arising in epidermal cyst (EC). The age at presentation ranged from 60 to 96 years. In all cases histological examination revealed a cyst lined by stratified squamous epithelium exhibiting keratinisation. The cystic epithelium showed in situ SCC *squamous cell carcinoma* in continuity with invasive keratinizing component. The study for HPV was negative. Perineal cystic nodule was found in a 86 year-old woman. The wall showed varying degrees of papillomatosis, hypergranulosis, parakeratosis with dysplastic and koilocytic changes. An invasive SCC *squamous cell carcinoma* was found in continuity with in situ malignant cystic epithelium. Using polymerase chain reaction and in situ hybridization, they have detected the presence of human papillomavirus (HPV) genotype 16 in the cystic wall and in the invasive carcinoma. CT scan showed a diffuse wall thickening of the anorectal region and infiltration of anus levators muscle. The histopathology examination of endoscopic biopsies of the anal canal and rectum revealed a SCC *squamous cell carcinoma* with presence of HPV 16. The patient refused any kind of treatment. The diagnosis of SCC arising from verrucous cyst (HPV associated cyst) was performed with extensive involvement of anal canal. A lesion may be diagnosed as "SCC arising in an EC" only with the support of an accurate histological documentation in order to exclude mimics (proliferating epidermoid cyst, proliferating trichilemmal cyst, and pseudocarcinomatous hyperplasia in a ruptured cyst). HPV demonstration has to be negative in order to exclude a verrucous cyst. The main histological feature essential for diagnosis is the presence of a "continuum" between cystic wall and SCC. Appling this diagnostic criterion many reported cases shouldn't been classified in this group. Despite the low risk of malignant transformation, it is generally agreed that all suspected cutaneous cysts should be submitted for histological examination. Regarding verrucous cyst, the site, the malignant transformation, the finding of HPV 16 type and the extensive neoplastic involvement of adjacent organ may be considered features of an extraordinary rare case.

In: Cysts: Causes, Diagnosis and Treatment Options
Editors: A. Mendes Ortiz and A. Jimenez Moreno

ISBN: 978-1-62081-315-7
© 2012 Nova Science Publishers, Inc.

Chapter 1

RECENT ADVANCES IN THE DIAGNOSTIC IMAGING OF CYSTS AND PSEUDOCYSTS IN THE ORAL AND MAXILLOFACIAL REGION

Jun-ichi Asaumi*, Hironobu Konouchi,
Yoshinobu Yanagi, Miki Hisatomi, Hidenobu Matsuzaki,
Jun Murakami, Teruhisa Unetsubo,
Mariko Fujita and Marina Hara
Department of Oral and Maxillofacial Radiology, Okayama University Graduate Schools
of Medicine, Dentistry and Pharmaceutical Sciences, Japan

ABSTRACT

It is sometimes difficult to differentiate cysts and pseudocysts from tumors in the jawbone on the basis of conventional radiographs. Moreover, cysts and pseudocysts that arise in soft tissue can not be detected on radiographic images without the use of contrast agents. Therefore, additional information is sometimes required to diagnose these lesions. Computed tomography and magnetic resonance imaging (CT; MRI) have been demonstrated to be very useful for depicting normal structures and pathological processes in the oral and maxillofacial region. Whereas CT is best for depicting bone structures, MRI is superior to CT at evaluating soft tissue. The contents of bone lesions might also be better visualized on MRI.

In this chapter, among the variety of lesions that occur in the oral and maxillofacial region, we would like to focus on those arising in the jaw or adjacent soft tissue. We present their representative CT and MRI findings and discuss the imaging characteristics that most contribute to their differential diagnosis.

1. Cysts and pseudocysts that affect the jaw

* Address correspondence to: Junichi Asaumi, Department of Oral and Maxillofacial Radiology, Field of Tumor Biology, Okayama University Graduate School of Medicine, Dentistry and Pharmaceutical Sciences, 5-1, Shikata-cho, 2-Chome, Kita-ku, Okayama 700-8558, Japan; E-mail: asaumi@md.okayama-u.ac.jp; Telephone number: +81-86-235-6705; Fax number: +81-86-235-6709.

        1-a True cysts
            1-a-1) Radicular cyst
            1-a-2) Dentigerous cyst
            1-a-3) Nasopalatine duct cyst
            1-a-4) Postoperative maxillary cyst
        1-b Pseudocysts
            1-b-1) Simple bone cyst
            1-b-2) Aneurysmal bone cyst
            1-b-3) Static bone cavity
   2.   Cysts that affect soft tissue
            2-1) Nasolabial cyst
            2-2) Mucous retention cyst
            2-3) Dermoid/epidermoid cyst
            2-4) Epidermal cyst
            2-5) Branchial cleft cyst
            2-6) Thyroglossal duct cyst
            2-7) Ranula
   3.   Others
            3-1) Keratocystic odontogenic tumor

INTRODUCTION

Many kinds of cystic lesion develop in the jawbone and adjacent soft tissue. These cystic lesions can be divided into true cysts, which have an epithelial lining, and pseudocysts, which do not have an epithelial lining, although the latter group also includes certain tumors. It is sometimes difficult to differentiate cysts and pseudocysts from tumors affecting the jaw on the basis of conventional radiographs. Moreover, cysts and pseudocysts that develop in soft tissue can not be detected on radiographic images without the use of contrast agents. Therefore, additional advanced information is sometimes required in order to diagnose these lesions. Computed tomography and magnetic resonance imaging (CT; MRI) have been demonstrated to be excellent for depicting normal structures and pathological processes in the oral and maxillofacial region. Whereas CT is best for depicting bony structures, MRI is superior to CT at evaluating soft tissue. The contents of bone lesions might also be better visualized on MRI because of the broad range of MRI sequences although the contents of cysts can also be represented using CT values.

In this chapter, among the wide variety of lesions that occur in the oral and maxillofacial region, we focus on cysts and pseudocysts that arise in the jawbone or adjacent soft tissue and keratocystic odontogenic tumor, which was previously classified as an odontogenic cyst. We present their representative CT and MR images and discuss the imaging characteristics that most contribute to their differential diagnosis.

1. CYSTS AND PSEUDOCYSTS THAT AFFECT THE JAW

1a. True Cysts

1a.1. Radicular Cyst

Radicular cysts are the most common type of cyst affecting the jaw [1]. They are also known as periapical cysts. Radicular cysts arise through the proliferation of epithelial tissue from the rests of Malassez within a periapical granuloma. This epithelial proliferation is triggered by inflammation secondary to pulpal necrosis following caries or trauma [2]. Most radicular cysts develop without symptoms, and they are often discovered when patients present with swelling and pain as their main complaints. Radicular cysts rarely recur after appropriate management [3].

Diagnostic Imaging

Radicular cysts appear as a round or oval area of radiolucency in the periapical region of the affected tooth (Figure 1a.1.1.). Loss of the lamina dura occurs along the adjacent root, and a rounded area of radiolucency encircles the affected tooth apex [3]. This finding is important for diagnosing radicular cysts, and intraoral radiographs are useful for detecting it (Figure 1a.1.2a.). Radicular cysts come in various sizes, are generally well delineated, and usually display a markedly radiopaque rim. Axial mandibular occlusal radiographs are useful for examinations of buccolingual swelling caused by mandibular radicular cysts (Figure 1a.1.2b).

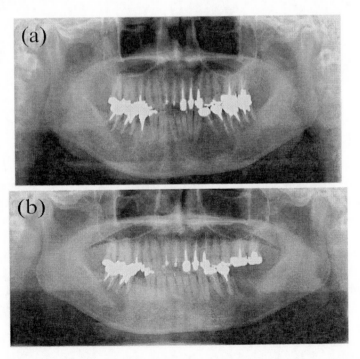

Figure 1a.1.1. Panoramic radiographs of a radicular cyst in a 33-year-old male. (a) A well-defined unilocular area of radiolucency associated with the apex of the left mandibular first premolar. (b) The patient is doing well 22 months after surgery.

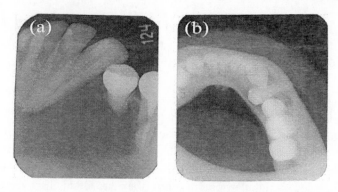

Figure 1a.1.2. Intraoral radiographs of a radicular cyst. (a) A periapical radiograph shows a unilocular area of radiolucency surrounding the periodontal space of the left mandibular first premolar. (b) A mandibular occlusal radiograph shows buccal expansion and lingual inclination of the left mandibular first premolar.

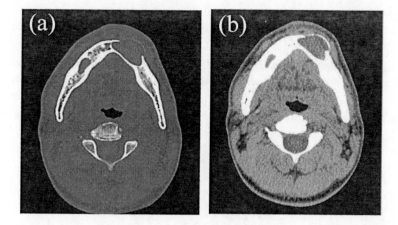

Figure 1a.1.3. CT images of radicular cysts. (a) An axial CT image obtained using the bone window shows buccal expansion with a sclerotic border. (b) A CT scan obtained using the soft tissue window displays a radiodensity of 30 HU, which is indicative of a water-like density.

The widely accepted early view of McCall and Wald was that radicular cysts could be radiographically differentiated from granulomas on the basis of their larger size (more than 9.5 mm in diameter) [4, 5]. Thus, if a lesion has a radiographic area of greater than 200 mm^2 or a greatest radiographic dimension of greater than 20 mm, it is considered to be a radicular cyst [6].

CT examinations are useful for diagnosing large radicular cysts, which almost always involve several teeth; revealing the relationship between the lesion and the surrounding tissue; and understanding the three-dimensional structure of the lesion. As radicular cysts increase in size, they have a tendency to undergo buccolingual expansion (Figure 1a.1.3a). Depending on the position of the lesion, CT scans can show deviation of the normal adjacent structures such as the mandibular canal, maxillary sinus floor, etc. When CT is performed using the soft tissue window, the interior regions of radicular cysts display CT values that are indicative of a water-like density (~30 HU) (Figure 1a.1.3b). Contrast-enhanced CT scans of radicular cysts shows rim-enhancement, but the inner part of the cyst is not enhanced.

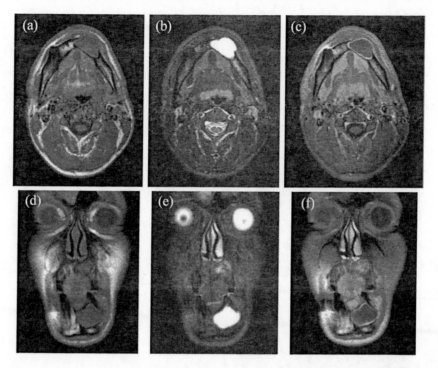

Figure 1a.1.4. MR images of radicular cysts. Radicular cysts display isointensity on axial T1WI (TR/TE=660/15) (a) and homogeneous hyperintensity on short TI inversion recovery (STIR) images (TR/TE=4500/60) (b). (c) On CE-T1WI (TR/TE=660/15), radicular cysts display rim-enhancement, and the inner part of the cyst is not enhanced. (d) Coronal T1WI (TR/TE=660/15), (e) STIR images (TR/TE=4500/60), and (f) CE-T1WI (TR/TE=660/15) show the same features as axial images.

Radicular cysts display a predilection for homogeneous isointensity on T1 weighted images (WI) and homogeneous hyperintensity on T2WI (Figure 1a.1.4a, 4b.). Contrast-enhanced T1WI demonstrate uniform isointensity and thin peripheral rim enhancement, but the cyst contents are not enhanced (Figure 1a.1.4c) [7-9]. Sometimes, radicular cysts show heterogeneous hypo- to hyperintensity on MR images, which could indicate that they have become infected and contain pus, seropurulent fluid, or sanguinopurulent fluid.

Dynamic contrast-enhanced MRI (DCE-MRI) are created from a series of MRI images and can be used to observe the flow pattern of contrast medium into a lesion (Figure 1a.1.5a) [9-12]. Regions of interest (ROI) are drawn by free hand drawing using a cursor on a monitor so that they include the cyst contents (ROI 1), the maximal region of the lesion, (ROI 2), and part of the cyst wall (ROI 3) (1a.1.5b). The signal intensity of each ROI is then plotted on a time course to obtain a time-signal intensity curve (Figure 1a.1.5c). The time-signal intensity curves of the cyst cavities (ROI 1) of radicular cysts are flat, whereas those for the maximal region of the lesion, which includes part of the cyst wall (ROI 2), and part of the cyst wall alone (ROI 3) gradually increase after the administration of Gd-DTPA. In summary, the cyst contents of radicular cysts are not enhanced, and their cyst walls display gradual enhancement. Although the maximal region of the lesion is often included in the ROI, DCE-MRI of cystic lesions such as radicular cysts (ROI 2) also reflect the enhancement of part of the cyst wall. Clinicians should recognize that radicular cysts only display partial enhancement.

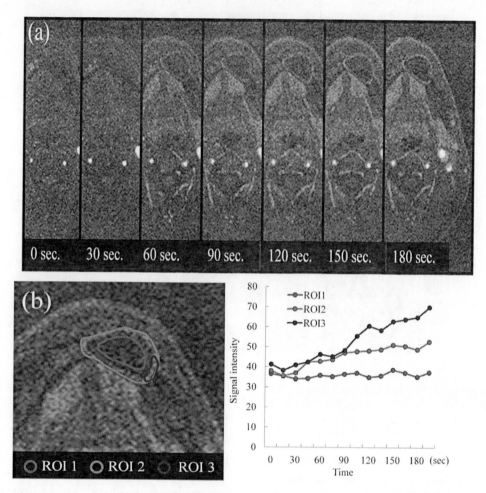

Figure 1a.1.5. DCE-MRI of radicular cysts. (a) A series of dynamic MR images showing the contrast medium flow pattern. (b) The region of interest (ROI) was drawn to include the inner part of the cyst (ROI 1), the maximal region of the lesion together with part of the cyst wall (ROI 2), and part of the cyst wall alone (ROI 3). (c) The signal intensity of each ROI was plotted on a time course to obtain a time-signal intensity curve.

Pathological Findings

Histologically, most radicular cysts are lined by a non-keratinized stratified squamous epithelium [1]. The morphology of the epithelium is dependent upon the degree of inflammation. Initially, it is usually thick, irregular, stratified, and squamous, but as it matures the lining becomes thinner and more regular, and the inflammation of the underlying cyst wall is usually less severe [2].

Radicular cysts usually contain a sterile straw-colored fluid with an iridescent sheen, which is imparted by cholesterol crystals [13]. Their contents are occasionally thick and caseous and include epithelial and hemorrhagic debris. More recent studies have shown that their cystic fluid is largely composed of inflammatory exudate; i.e., it contains several high molecular weight proteins, and low weight proteins are present in similar concentrations to those found in plasma. The fluid also contains other inflammatory exudate components including cholesterol, erythrocyte and inflammatory cell breakdown products, epithelial cells, and fibrin [3].

REFERENCES

[1]   IRH Kramer, JJ Pindborg, M Shear. *Histological Typirg of Odontogenic Tumours.* 2nd edition. Springer-Verlag, Berlin Heidelberg, 1992.

[2]   Roderick A Cawson, W.H. Binnie, Andrew W. Barrett, John M. Wright. *Oral Disease,* 3rd edition. Mosby, 2001.

[3]   Neville BW, Damm DD, Allen CM, Bouquot JE. *Oral and Maxillofacial Pathology,* 2nd edition. Philadelphia: WB Saunders Co, 2002.

[4]   McCall JO, Wald SS. *Clinical dental roentgenology.* 3rd edition. Philadelphia: WB Saunders Co.; 1952.

[5]   Natkin E, Oswald RJ, Carnes LI. The relationship of lesion size to diagnosis, incidence, and treatment of periapical cysts and granulomas. *Oral Surg Oral Med Oral Pathol* 1984;57:82-94.

[6]   Zain RB, Roswati N, Ismail K. Radiographic evaluation of lesion sizes of histologically diagnosed periapical cysts and granulomas. *Ann Dent* 1989;48:3-5, 46.

[7]   Hisatomi M, Asaumi J, Konouchi H, Shigehara H, Yanagi Y, Kishi K. MR imaging of epithelial cysts of the oral and maxillofacial region. *Eur J Radiol* 2003;48:178-82.

[8]   Minami M, Kaneda T, Ozawa K, Yamamoto H, Itai Y, Ozawa M, Yoshikawa K, Sasaki Y. Cystic lesions of the maxillomandibular region: MR imaging distinction of odontogenic keratocysts and ameloblastomas from other cysts. *AJR Am J Roentgenol* 1996;166:943-9.

[9]   Yanagi Y, Asaumi J, Unetsubo T, Ashida M, Takenobu T, Hisatomi M, Matsuzaki H, Konouchi H, Katase N, Nagatsuka H. Usefulness of MRI and dynamic contrast-enhanced MRI for differential diagnosis of simple bone cysts from true cysts in the jaw. *Oral Surg Oral Med Oral Pathol Oral Radiol Endod* 2010;110:364-9.

[10] Hisatomi M, Yanagi Y, Konouchi H, Matsuzaki H, Takenobu T, Unetsubo T, Asaumi J. Diagnostic value of dynamic contrast-enhanced MRI for unilocular cystic-type ameloblastomas with homogeneously bright high signal intensity on T2-weighted or STIR MR images. *Oral Oncol* 2011;47:147-52.

[11] Unetsubo T, Konouchi H, Yanagi Y, Murakami J, Fujii M, Matsuzaki H, Hisatomi M, Nagatsuka H, Asaumi JI. Dynamic contrast-enhanced magnetic resonance imaging for estimating tumor proliferation and microvessel density of oral squamous cell carcinomas. *Oral Oncol* 2009;45:621-6.

[12] Hisatomi M, Asaumi JI, Yanagi Y, Unetsubo T, Maki Y, Murakami J, Matsuzaki H, Honda Y, Konouchi H. Diagnostic value of dynamic contrast-enhanced MRI in the salivary gland tumors. *Oral Oncol* 2007;43:940-7.

[13] Archer WH. *Oral and maxillofacial surgery,* 5th edition. Philadelphia: WB Saunders Co, 1975.

1a.2. Dentigerous Cyst

Dentigerous cysts are single cysts that enclose the crown of an unerupted tooth [1-3]. They develop via the accumulation of fluid between the reduced enamel epithelium and the crown, or between the layers of the reduced enamel epithelium [3]. There are two types of dentigerous cyst, the developmental and inflammatory types [4]. The first type is developmental in origin and occurs in mature teeth, usually as a result of impaction. The second type is inflammatory in origin and occurs in immature teeth as a result of inflammation in a non-vital deciduous tooth. Alternatively, inflammation can occur in another tissue and then subsequently spread to a nearby tooth follicle [4, 5].

Diagnostic Imaging

Radiographically, dentigerous cysts appear as a well-defined unilocular radiolucent area associated with the crown of an unerupted tooth (Figure 1a.2.1.). Radiographic findings are useful for diagnosing typical dentigerous cysts as their borders are continuous with the cementoenamel junction of the impacted tooth.

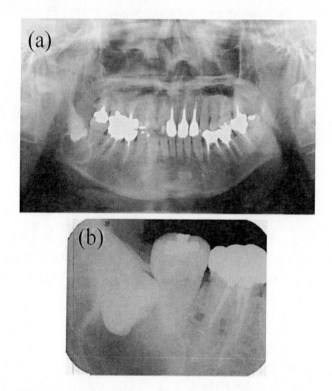

Figure 1a.2.1. A typical dentigerous cyst in a 45-year-old male. (a) A panoramic radiograph shows a well-defined radiolucent area associated with the crown of an impacted right third molar. (b) A periapical radiograph demonstrates that the dentigerous cyst has expanded in the follicle and become attached to the cementoenamel junction of the unerupted tooth.

Dentigerous cysts are most often found in association with a mandibular third molar, maxillary canine, or third molar, followed by a mandibular second premolar [3]. Clinicians should also be aware that dentigerous cysts sometimes affect mesiodens teeth (Figure 1a.2.2.) [6-8]. Asaumi et al. reported that dentigerous cysts arising from mesiodens teeth accounted for 22 of 200 dentigerous cyst cases (11%) [7]. Dentigerous cysts that involve premolars are often seen during the mixed dentition period [5, 9, 10]. Most dentigerous cysts that arise during this period are of the inflammatory type, and deciduous teeth that have been treated with root canal therapy and those with severe caries are at risk of dentigerous cyst development. The radiographic findings of inflammatory dentigerous cysts include a unilocular area of radiolucency that appears to include the apical side of an incomplete permanent tooth and extends beyond the cementoenamel junction, sometimes involving the entire root. It is generally accepted that extraction of a non-vital primary tooth and marsupialization allow rapid healing of the lesion and eruption of the permanent tooth, provided that these procedures are performed during the normal eruption period [4, 11].

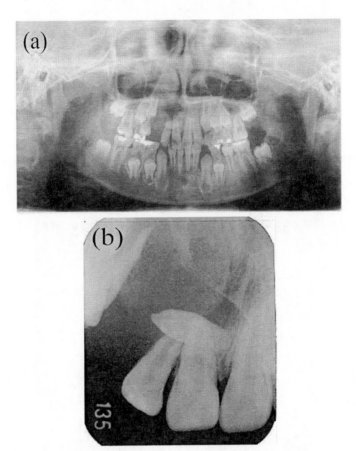

Figure 1a.2.2. A dentigerous cyst in a 9-year-old male. (a) A panoramic radiograph shows a radiolucent area associated with a mesiodens in the right anterior region. (b) The lesion appeared to involve the mesiodens on a periapical radiograph.

Although typical dentigerous cyst radiographs display a round well-defined cavity enclosing a tooth crown, panoramic and/or periapical radiographs are inadequate for showing the relationship between the cyst and the cementoenamel junction when the associated tooth is impacted in the buccolingual direction. Thus, reconstructed CT images are useful for examining the relationship between the cyst and the associated tooth. CT might contribute to the definitive diagnosis of dentigerous cysts in cases that are difficult to diagnose on panoramic and/or periapical radiographs (Figure 1a.2.3.).

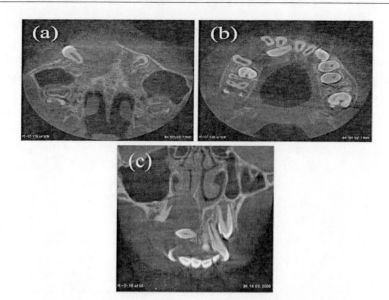

Figure 1a.2.3. A dentigerous cyst in a 9-year-old male. (a) An axial image obtained with cone-beam CT shows a unilocular radiolucent area in the right anterior area. (b) Cone-beam CT obtained at the level of a mesiodens shows that the dentigerous cyst is associated with the crown of the mesiodens. (c) On a reconstructed coronal CT image, the lesion displayed an expansive appearance and had elevated the floor of the nasal cavity.

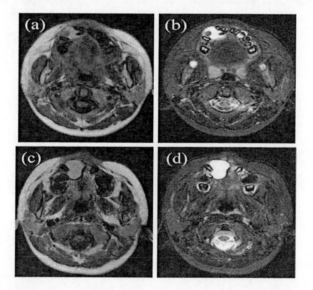

Figure 1a.2.4. A dentigerous cyst in a 9-year-old male. MR images taken at the level of a mesiodens showing a dentigerous cyst associated with the crown of the mesiodens ((a) T1WI, (b) STIR image). The dentigerous cyst displays hyperintensity on axial T1WI (TR/TE=540/15) (c) and homogeneous hyperintensity on short TI inversion recovery (STIR) images (TR/TE=6100/60) (d).

Dentigerous cysts tend to display homogeneous hyperintensity on T2WI and demonstrate a variety of signal intensities ranging from homogeneous hypo- to hyperintensity on T1WI (Figure Figure 1a.2.4) [12, 13]. As dentigerous cysts have many opportunities to become infected or bleed, many dentigerous cysts show modified hyperintensity on T1WI. Contrast-enhanced T1WI of these cysts display a thin peripheral rim enhancement.

Pathological Findings

Histologically, the cyst wall is composed of a thin layer of connective tissue lined by an epithelium that might only be two to three non-keratinized stratified squamous cells thick [1-3]. The epithelium is contiguous with the reduced enamel epithelium at the cementoenamel junction.

If inflammation is present, inflammatory changes are sometimes seen in fibrous connective tissue, and the epithelium displays elongated rete pegs. Desquamated epithelial cells and blood components can fall into the cystic cavity. (see Japanese Dental Science Review 2011; in press)

References

[1]   Neville BW, Damm DD, Allen CM, Bouquot JE. *Oral and Maxillofacial Pathology*, 2nd edition. Philadelphia: WB Saunders Co, 2002.

[2]   Roderick A Cawson, W.H. Binnie, Andrew W. Barrett, John M. *Wright. Oral Disease*, 3rd edition. Mosby, 2001.

[3]   IRH Kramer, JJ Pindborg, M Shear. *Histological Typirg of Odontogenic Tumours*. 2nd edition. Springer-Verlag, Berlin Heidelberg, 1992.

[4]   Benn A, Altini M. Dentigerous cysts of inflammatory origin. A clinicopathologic study. *Oral Surg Oral Med Oral Pathol Oral Radiol Endod* 1996;81:203–209.

[5]   Shibata Y, Asaumi J, Yanagi Y, Kawai N, Hisatomi M, Matsuzaki H, Konouchi H, Nagatsuka H, Kishi K. Radiographic examination of dentigerous cysts in the transitional dentition. *Dentomaxillofac Radiol* 2004;33:17-20.

[6]   Lustmann J, Bodner L. Dentigerous cysts associated with supernumerary teeth. *Int J Oral Maxillofac Surg* 1988;17:100-2.

[7]   Asaumi JI, Shibata Y, Yanagi Y, Hisatomi M, Matsuzaki H, Konouchi H, Kishi K. Radiographic examination of mesiodens and their associated complications. *Dentomaxillofac Radiol* 2004;33:125-7.

[8]   Som PM, Shangold LM, Biller HF. A palatal dentigerous cyst arising from a mesiodente. *AJNR Am J Neuroradiol* 1992;13:212-4.

[9]   Yahara Y, Kubota Y, Yamashiro T, Shirasuna K. Eruption prediction of mandibular premolars associated with dentigerous cysts. *Oral Surg Oral Med Oral Pathol Oral Radiol Endod* 2009;108:28-31.

[10] Fujii R, Kawakami M, Hyomoto M, Ishida J, Kirita T. Panoramic findings for predicting eruption of mandibular premolars associated with dentigerous cyst after marsupialization. *J Oral Maxillofac Surg* 2008;66:272-6.

[11] Takagi S, Koyama S. Guided eruption of an impacted second premolar associated with a dentigerous cyst in the maxillary sinus of a 6-year-old child. *J Oral Maxillofac Surg* 1998;56:237-9.

[12] Hisatomi M, Asaumi J, Konouchi H, Shigehara H, Yanagi Y, Kishi K. MR imaging of epithelial cysts of the oral and maxillofacial region. *Eur J Radiol* 2003;48:178-82.

[13] Konouchi H, Yanagi Y, Hisatomi M, Matsuzaki H, Takenobu T, Unetsubo T, Asaumi J., *MR image diagnostic protocol for unilocular lesions of the jaws*. Japanese Dental Science Review 2011 in press.

1a.3. Nasopalatine Duct Cyst

Nasopalatine duct cyst is a common developmental nonodontogenic cyst affecting the oral cavity. Although the pathogenesis of this lesion remains uncertain, it probably results from the spontaneous cystic degeneration of remnants of the nasopalatine duct [1, 2]. Asymptomatic lesions of less than 6 mm in diameter are regarded as enlarged incisor ducts [1, 3, 4]. Many incisive canals contain 1 inferior foramen and 2 superior foramina, and the separating level is located just beneath the nasal floor (Figure 1a.3.1) [5]. Bilateral nasopalatine duct cysts occasionally develop at certain sites [6].

Diagnostic Imaging

Radiographs of nasopalatine duct cysts usually demonstrate a well-circumscribed area of radiolucency on or near the midline of the anterior maxilla between the apical and central incisor teeth. Some cysts show a classic heart shape as a result of the superimposition of the nasal spine or because they have been notched by the nasal septum [1]. Sometimes it is difficult to differentiate nasopalatine duct cysts from radicular cysts. The preservation of the periodontal spaces of the maxillary central incisor teeth and the separation of the apex of the right maxillary central incisor from that of the left maxillary central incisor are useful findings for differentiating nasopalatine duct cysts from radicular cysts. Intraoral radiographs should be used for diagnosing nasopalatine duct cysts because the shadow of the cervical vertebrae, which often disturbs the clarity of the anterior region, is present on panoramic radiographs.

The characteristic CT findings of nasopalatine cysts are a midline location, smooth expansion with sclerotic margins, and tooth apex displacement. Radicular cysts differ in that the teeth apices are within the cyst rather than being displaced [7]. Coronal and/or sagittal reconstructed CT images of nasopalatine cysts display expansion of the incisive canal (Figure 1a.3.2), and reconstructed CT images are useful for demonstrating the buccolingual expansion of the lesion and its the relationship with the nasal floor.

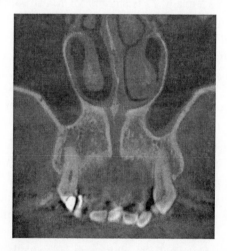

Figure 1a.3.1. Reconstructed cone-beam CT image of an incisive canal in a 37-year-old female. The incisive canal has 1 inferior foramen and 2 superior foramina, and the separating level is located just beneath the nasal floor.

Diagnostic Imaging

Radiographs of nasopalatine duct cysts usually demonstrate a well-circumscribed area of radiolucency on or near the midline of the anterior maxilla between the apical and central incisor teeth. Some cysts show a classic heart shape as a result of the superimposition of the nasal spine or because they have been notched by the nasal septum [1]. Sometimes it is difficult to differentiate nasopalatine duct cysts from radicular cysts. The preservation of the periodontal spaces of the maxillary central incisor teeth and the separation of the apex of the right maxillary central incisor from that of the left maxillary central incisor are useful findings for differentiating nasopalatine duct cysts from radicular cysts. Intraoral radiographs should be used for diagnosing nasopalatine duct cysts because the shadow of the cervical vertebrae, which often disturbs the clarity of the anterior region, is present on panoramic radiographs.

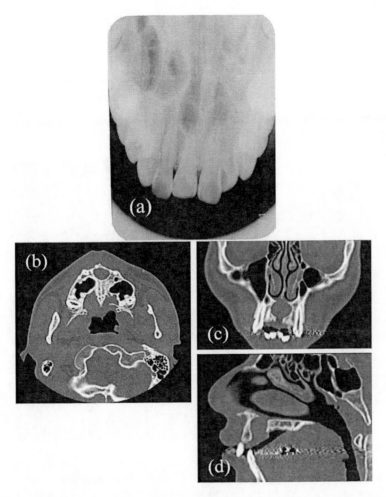

Figure 1a.3.2. A nasopalatine duct cyst in a 21-year-old male. (a) An occlusal radiograph showing a well-demarcated area of radiolucency located on the midline of the palate, apical to the central incisor teeth. The periodontal spaces of the central incisor teeth have been preserved. (b) An axial CT image demonstrated a round radiolucent area with a greatest diameter of 17 mm located on the palatal midline. (c) A coronal reconstructed CT image demonstrated destruction of the nasal floor and expansion of the incisive canal. (d) A sagittal reconstructed CT image showed a well-defined mass that extended to the palate.

The characteristic CT findings of nasopalatine cysts are a midline location, smooth expansion with sclerotic margins, and tooth apex displacement. Radicular cysts differ in that the teeth apices are within the cyst rather than being displaced [7]. Coronal and/or sagittal reconstructed CT images of nasopalatine cysts display expansion of the incisive canal (Figure 1a.3.2), and reconstructed CT images are useful for demonstrating the buccolingual expansion of the lesion and its the relationship with the nasal floor.

MR images of nasopalatine duct cysts tend to show homogeneous hyperintensity on both T1WI and T2WI (Figure 1a.3.3) [8, 9]. Some nasopalatine duct cysts have been reported to show homogeneous isointensity on T1WI [10, 11]. Contrast-enhanced T1WI show enhancement of the lesion rim. The cyst contents are not enhanced.

Pathological Findings

The epithelial linings of nasopalatine duct cysts are highly variable. They can be composed of a stratified squamous epithelium, pseudostratified columnar epithelium, simple columnar epithelium, or simple cuboidal epithelium [1, 2]. The type of epithelium depends on the location of the cyst and might also reflect the pluripotential character of the embryonic epithelial remnants [12]. Cysts developing within the superior aspect of the canal near the nasal cavity are more likely to include a respiratory epithelium, whereas those located in an inferior position near the oral cavity are more likely to exhibit a squamous epithelium.

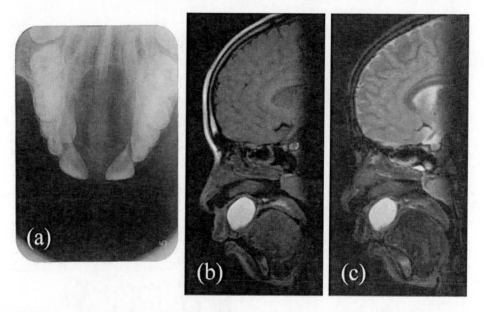

Figure 1a.3.3. A nasopalatine duct cyst in a 7-year-old male. (a) An occlusal radiograph showing a lesion with a diameter of 25 mm, which appeared as an ovoid area of radiolucency located on the midline of the maxilla. The lesion displayed homogeneous hyperintensity on both T1WI ((b) TR/TE=660/15) and T2WI ((c) TR/TE=3000/90). Adapted from reference no.8 (Hisatomi M et al. MR imaging of epithelial cysts of the oral and maxillofacial region. Eur J Radiol. 2003;48:178-82. doi:10.1016/S0720-048X(02)00218-8)

References

[1]   Neville BW, Damm DD, Allen CM, Bouquot JE. *Oral and Maxillofacial Pathology,* 2nd edition. Philadelphia: WB Saunders Co, 2002.

[2]   Kramer IRH, Pindborg JJ, Shear M. *Histological Typirg of Odontogenic Tumours.* 2nd edition. Springer-Verlag, Berlin Heidelberg, 1992.

[3]   Swanson KS, Kaugars GE, Gunsolley JC. Nasopalatine duct cyst: an analysis of 334 cases. *J Oral Maxillofac Surg* 1991;49:268-71.

[4]   Vasconcelos R, De Aguiar MF, Castro W, De Araújo VC, Mesquita R. Retrospective analysis of 31 cases of nasopalatine duct cyst. Oral Dis 1999;5:325-8.

[5]   Song WC, Jo DI, Lee JY, Kim JN, Hur MS, Hu KS, Kim HJ, Shin C, Koh KS. Microanatomy of the incisive canal using three-dimensional reconstruction of microCT images: an ex vivo study. *Oral Surg Oral Med Oral Pathol Oral Radiol Endod* 2009;108:583-90.

[6]   Cicciù M, Grossi GB, Borgonovo A, Santoro G, Pallotti F, Maiorana C. Rare bilateral nasopalatine duct cysts: a case report. *Open Dent J* 2010;4:8-12.

[7]   Pevsner PH, Bast WG, Lumerman H, Pivawer G. CT analysis of a complicated nasopalatine duct cyst. *N Y State Dent J* 2000;66:18-20.

[8]   Hisatomi M, Asaumi J, Konouchi H, Shigehara H, Yanagi Y, Kishi K. MR imaging of epithelial cysts of the oral and maxillofacial region. *Eur J Radiol* 2003;48:178-82. doi:10.1016/S0720-048X(02)00218-8.

[9]   Hisatomi M, Asaumi J, Konouchi H, Matsuzaki H, Kishi K. MR imaging of nasopalatine duct cysts. *Eur J Radiol* 2001;39:73-6. doi:10.1016/S0720-048X(01) 00279-0.

[10] Tanaka S, Iida S, Murakami S, Kishino M, Yamada C, Okura M. Extensive nasopalatine duct cyst causing nasolabial protrusion. *Oral Surg Oral Med Oral Pathol Oral Radiol Endod* 2008;106:e46-50.

[11] Robertson H, Palacios E. Nasopalatine duct cyst. *Ear Nose Throat* J 2004;83:313.

[12] Shafer WG, Hine MK, Levy BM. *A textbook of oral pathology.* 3rd edition. Philadelphia: WB Saunders Co, 1974.

1a.4. Postoperative Maxillary Cyst

Postoperative maxillary cysts (POMC) were first reported by Kubo in 1927 [1] as a maxillary cyst that arose after surgical treatment for maxillary sinusitis. POMC appear as tumors associated with sinus bone expansion and can have a unilocular or multilocular structure. In English, Gregory and Shafer [2] first reported these cystic lesions as "surgical ciliated cysts of the maxilla". They are also known as "secondary mucocele" [3, 4], "paranasal cysts", or "maxillary sinus mucocele" [5-8]. Many cases have been reported. Although POMC is quite rare in the West, it is more common in Asia [9, 10]. The largest series of cases have been reported in Asian populations, especially in Japan. In Japan, POMC is one of the most common maxillary cysts, where it constitutes 20% of all oral cysts [11-14]. POMC occurs as a delayed complication many years after surgical intervention in the maxillary sinus, e.g., after midface osteotomy, midfacial fractures, gunshot injuries, the Caldwell-Luc procedure, and raising of the sinus floor [15-18]. The patient's initial complaint often involves pain, swelling, and drainage in the buccal region [11, 16]. Gradually, the lesion expands beyond the original sinus boundaries, resulting in perforation of the sinus wall. It presents as an expansile swelling of the cheek or palate. A history of maxillary surgical intervention is also important for obtaining a diagnosis of POMC. Enucleation or marsupialization of the cyst is considered to be effective for the treatment of POMC [19]. POMC is believed to result from entrapment of the sinus and/or nasal mucosa in the wound during closure after the Caldwell-Luc procedure [1, 11, 12, 20]. During the healing phase, the entrapped sinonasal mucosa proliferates and creates a ciliated cyst. Histologically, the cyst is usually lined with a pseudostratified ciliated columnar epithelium of the respiratory type, but transition to a columnar, cuboidal, or even squamous epithelium has also been reported [11].

Radiographically, it appears as a well-defined unilocular or multilocular area of radiolucency in the maxillary sinus, and in some instances it causes bony perforation. On panoramic radiographs, it appears as a unilocular area of cystic radiolucency with well-defined lobular margins in the left maxillary sinus region (Figure 1a.4.1a). The lesion does not involve the neighboring teeth. Waters view radiographs have a limited ability to distinguish the lesion due to the superimposition of anatomic structures (Figure 1a.4.1b).

CT is the most useful method for diagnosing POMC and selecting an appropriate surgical approach. POMC display characteristic CT findings of localized bone defects and bulging. Figure 1.a.4.2a shows a homogenous cyst-like lesion (a POMC) that completely occupies the left maxillary sinus. It has eroded the inner and lateral walls of the maxillary sinus and expanded into the nasal cavity and cheek. On Ct images obtained with the bone window, it can be seen that the sinus wall has become thin and perforated (Figure 1a.4.2b). The lesion has also damaged the boundaries of the sinus, even perforating the nasal floor (Figure 1a.4.2d). CT clearly demonstrates that the lesion has been compartmentalized by bony septa. The contents of the cyst do not display contrast enhancement on contrast enhanced (CE) CT (Figure 1a.4.2c).

Consequently, MRI is also considered to be a powerful imaging modality for POMC as it is able to illustrate the cystic contents and borders of POMC. However, there are few reports about the MR findings of POMC [5, 10]. Han et al. [5] reported 4 cases of multilocular POMC that displayed different signal intensities in each compartment in 3 cases and extreme hyperintensity on both T1WI and T2WI in one case. Isoda et al. [10] examined 32 POMC with MR imaging and found that they displayed iso- or hyperintensity on T1WI. On T2WI, the POMC were classified into the hyperintensity type and the ring-like type, which displayed a hyperintense rim.

The POMC shown in Figure 1a.4.3 displayed a lobular and clear border, non-homogeneous isointensity on T1WI (Figure 1a.4.3a), and non-homogeneous hyperintensity on short TI inversion recovery (STIR) images (Figure 1a.4.3b). T1WI revealed that the contents of the lesion displayed isointensity to muscle. Furthermore, the interior of the lesion displayed homogeneous hyperintensity on T1WI and hypointensity on STIR images (Figure 1a.4.3a, b, d, e). The cyst did not display enhancement on CE-T1WI obtained with the fat saturation technique (Figure 1a.4.3c, f).

Chindasombatjaroen et al. [21] reported that most POMC displayed isointensity on T1WI and hyperintensity or non-homogeneous iso- and hyperintensity on T2WI obtained with the fat saturation technique. POMC tend to display a smooth border, and their contents do not display contrast medium enhancement on CT or MR images.

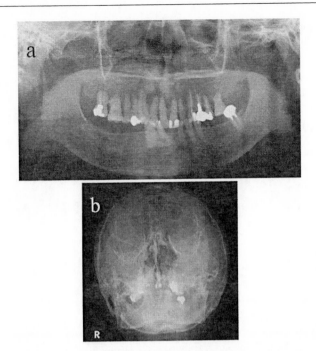

Figure 1a.4.1. (a) A panoramic radiograph (69-year-old female) showing a unilocular area of cystic radiolucency with well-defined lobular margins in the left maxillary sinus region. (b) Waters view radiographs have a limited ability to depict such lesions due to the superimposition of anatomical structures.

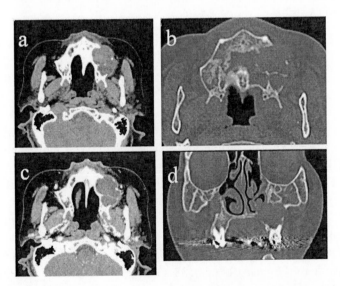

Figure 1a.4.2. (a-c) Axial CT images (69-year-old female) obtained before and after contrast medium administration. (a) An axial CT image obtained with the soft tissue window before contrast medium administration. A cyst was detected in the left maxillary sinus. The lesion had expanded beyond the original sinus boundaries. (b) Bone window CT revealed that the sinus wall had thinned and been perforated. The CT image clearly shows that the lesion has been compartmentalized by bony septa. (c) An axial CT image obtained after contrast medium administration. The contents of the cyst did not display contrast enhancement. (d) A reconstructed coronal image revealed that the lesion had damaged the boundaries of the sinus, resulting in perforation of the nasal floor.

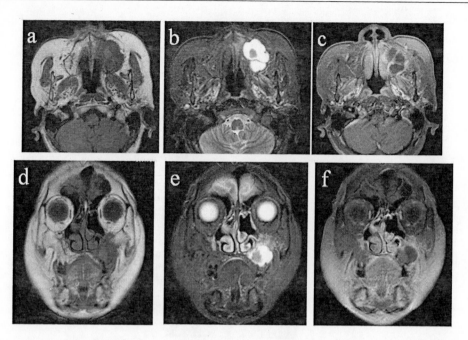

Figure 1a.4.3. MR images obtained before and after contrast medium administration (69-year-old female). (a, d) On T1WI, the lesion showed non-homogeneous isointensity to muscle. (b, e) On short TI inversion recovery images, the lesion displayed non-homogeneous hyperintensity a lobular structure and a clear border. The inside of the lesion appeared homogeneously hyperintense on T1WI and hypointense on STIR images. (c, f) T1WI obtained after contrast medium administration. Whist the rim was enhanced, the inner parts of the cyst were not.

The CT and MR findings of POMC patients can play powerful roles in reaching a diagnosis.

References

[1]   Kubo I. A buccal cyst occurred after radical operation of the maxillary sinus. *Z Otol Tokyo* 1927;39:896-7.

[2]   Gregory GT, Shafer WG. Surgical ciliated cysts of the maxilla. *J Oral Surg* 1958;16:251-3.

[3]   Som PM, Shugar JMA. Antral mucoceles: a new look. *J Comput Assist Tomogr* 1980;4:484-8.

[4]   Gardner DG, Gullane PJ. Mucoceles of the maxillary sinus. *Oral Surg Oral Med Oral Pathol Oral Radiol Endod* 1986;62:538-43.

[5]   Han MH, Chang KH, Lee CH, Na DG, Yeon KM, Han MC. Cystic expansile masses of the maxilla: differential diagnosis with CT and MR. *AJNR Am J Neuroradiol* 1995;16:333-8.

[6]   Thio D, Phelps PD, Bath AP. Maxillary sinus mucocele presenting as a late complication of a maxillary advancement procedure. *J Laryngol Otol* 2003;117:402-3.

[7]   Tsang RK, Woo JK, Van Hasselt CA. Compartmentalized maxillary sinus mucocele. *J Laryngol Otol* 1999;113:1106-8.

[8]   Billing KJ, Davis G, Selva D, Wilscek G, Mitchell R. Post-traumatic maxillary mucocele. *Ophthalmic Surg Lasers Imaging* 2004;35:152-5.

[9]   Hasegawa M, Saito Y, Watanabe I, Kern EB. Postoperative mucoceles of the maxillary sinus. *Rhinology* 1979;17:253-6.

[10] Isoda H, Takehara Y, Masui T, Seki A, Takahashi M, Kaneko M. MRI of postoperative maxillary cysts. *J Comput Assist Tomogr* 1993;17:572-5.

[11] Kaneshiro S, Nakajima T, Yoshikawa Y. The postoperative maxillary cyst: report of 71 cases. *J Oral Surg* 1981;39(3):191-8.

[12] Yamamoto H, Takagi M. Clinicopathologic study of the postoperative maxillary cyst. *Oral Surg Oral Med Oral Pathol* 1986;62(5):544-8.

[13] Maruyama M, Onodera K, Ooya K. A histopathological and lectin-histochemical study of the lining epithelium in postoperative maxillary cysts. *Oral Dis* 2002;8(5):241-8.

[14] Maeda Y, Osaki T, Yoneda K, Hirota J. Clinico-pathologic studies on post-operative maxillary cysts. *Int J Oral Maxillofac Surg* 1987;16(6):682-7.

[15] Amin M, Witherow H, Lee R, Blenkinsopp P. Surgical ciliated cyst after maxillary orthognathic surgery: report of a case. *J Oral Maxillofac Surg* 2003;61:138-41.

[16] Basu MK, Rout PG, Rippin JW, Smith AJ. Maxillary cyst: experience with 23 cases. *Int J Oral Maxillofac Surg* 1988;17:282-4.

[17] Sugar AW, Walker DM, Bounds GA. Surgical ciliated (postoperative maxillary) cysts following mid-face osteomies. *Br J Oral Maxillofac Surg* 1990;28:264-7.

[18] Lockhardt R, Ceccaldi J, Bertrand JC. Postoperative maxillary cyst following sinus bone graft: report of a case. *Int J Oral Maxillofac Implants* 2000;15:583-6.

[19] Yoshikawa Y, Nakajima T, Kaneshiro S, Sakaguchi M. Effective treatment of the postoperative maxillary cyst by marsupialization. *J Oral Maxillofac Surg* 1982;40(8):487-91.

[20] Tachikawa J. Clinico-pathological study of postoperative maxillary cyst. *J Tokyo Dent College Soc* 1975;75:1117-42.

[21] Chindasombatjaroen J, Uchiyama Y, Kakimoto N, Murakami S, Furukawa S, Kishino M. Postoperative maxillary cysts: magnetic resonance imaging compared with computerized tomography. *Oral Surg Oral Med Oral Pathol Oral Radiol Endod* 2009;107(5):e38-44.

1b. Pseudocysts

1b.1. Simple Bone Cyst

Simple bone cyst is classified as a bone-related lesion. The WHO defines simple bone cysts as 'intraosseous pseudocysts that are devoid of an epithelial lining and are either empty or filled with serous or sanguineous fluid' [1], and they have many synonyms, e.g., solitary bone cyst, traumatic bone cyst, hemorrhagic cyst, extravasation cyst, unicameral bone cyst, traumatic bone cyst, and idiopathic bone cavity, which might reflect our lack of knowledge about their etiology. Although several etiologic hypotheses have been proposed, the etiology of simple bone cysts remains a matter of conjecture. Among the abovementioned hypotheses, trauma is the most frequently discussed etiological factor. Simple bone cysts are not true cysts because they lack an epithelial lining and contain serous or sanguineous fluid in their cavities. In the maxillofacial region, simple bone cysts are commonly located in the body or symphysis of the mandible and are rarely seen in the maxilla. They are found in patients of all ages, but typically occur in adolescents and younger adults in their first to second decade of life without a significant gender predilection.

Radiographically, a scalloped appearance is a characteristic finding of this lesion. Most simple bone cysts are unilocular and have a clear margin. Sclerotic rims are unusual. Simple bone cysts often extend between tooth roots without causing displacement or resorption. They sometimes display cortical thinning and cortical bone expansion and dislocate the mandibular canal. CT scans reveal a unilocular low-density area with a clear border, and the density of the inner part of the lesion is equivalent to that of serum. A high-density area is sometimes seen within the lesion due to blood products degeneration or calcification.

Although most simple bone cysts can be diagnosed by conventional X-p and CT, they can be difficult to diagnose in cases that occur at unusual locations or show atypical radiographic features. In such cases, dynamic contrast-enhanced MRI is useful for obtaining additional information [2, 3]. On plain MRI, typical simple bone cysts display homogeneous iso- to slight hyperintensity on T1WI and homogeneous hyper- to marked hyperintensity on T2WI [2-5]. Some simple bone cysts show slightly heterogeneous signal intensities on both T1- and T2-WI. In these cases, the signal intensity varies depending on the age of the blood products contained in the cyst. On contrast-enhanced MRI, the periphery of the lesion is enhanced, as is seen in rim enhancement, and the inner part of the lesion displays slight enhancement [2, 3]. On dynamic contrast-enhanced MRI, a characteristic finding of simple bone cysts is gradual enhancement of the inner part of the lesion. The cavities of simple bone cysts are always filled with fluid [6], and the surrounding intramedullary fluid, which contains contrast agent, might exude into the cystic cavity through the peripheral fibrous connective tissue. The enhancement of the inner part of the lesion can take several minutes because intramedullary fluid flows very slowly. Thus, to confirm which areas have been enhanced by contrast medium injection, contrast-enhanced MR images must be acquired at least several minutes after the administration of the contrast agent, and the enhancement becomes stronger over time.

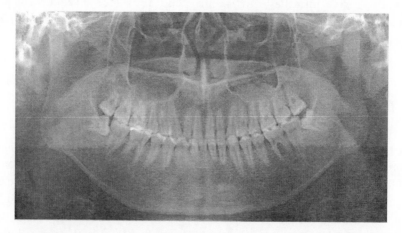

Figure 1b.1.1. A panoramic radiograph of a simple bone cyst in a 17-year-old male patient. The panoramic radiograph shows an ellipsoid, well-defined, lucent lesion that is undulating between the second molar and third molar teeth on the left side of the mandible. No tooth displacement or loss of the lamina dura of the roots had occurred. All of the patient's teeth were vital.

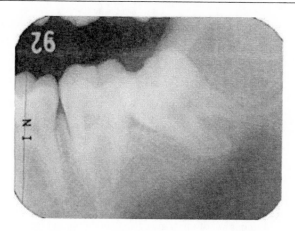

Figure 1b.1.2. Periapical radiograph of the same patient as shown in Figure 1b.1.1. The periapical radiograph clearly demonstrates that the lesion extends into the interdental space and does not have a sclerotic rim.

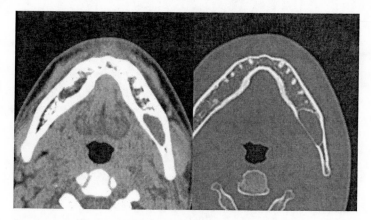

Figure 1b.1.3. CT images of the same patient as shown in Figure 1b.1.1. An axial CT scan showing an area of low attenuation on the left aspect of the mandible and thinning of the lingual cortex without expansion.

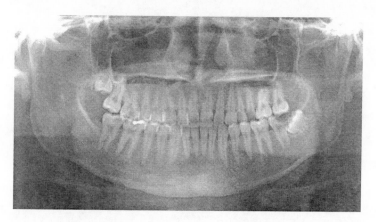

Figure 1b.1.4. Panoramic radiograph of simple bone cyst in a 19-year-old male patient. Panoramic radiograph shows an ill-defined, lucent lesion between the left and the right canine of the mandible.

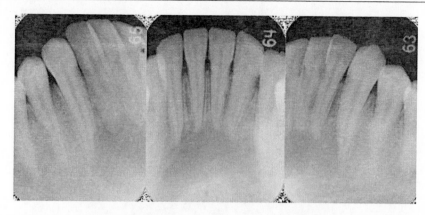

Figure 1b.1.5. A periapical radiograph of the same patient as shown in Figure 1b.1.4. The periapical radiograph clearly demonstrates that the lesion extends into the interdental space and does not have a sclerotic rim.

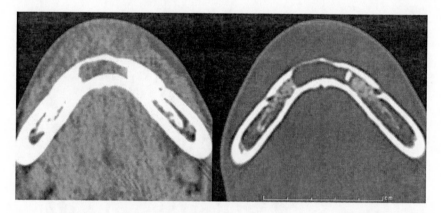

Figure 1b.1.6. CT images of the same patient as shown in Figure 1b.1.4. An axial CT scan shows an area of low attenuation in the center of the mandible. Slight expansion and cortical thinning are observed on the right labial side of the lesion.

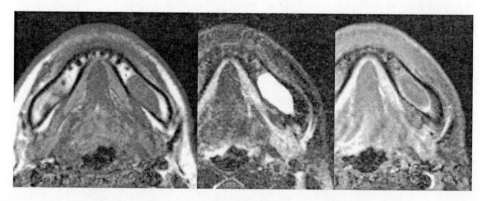

Figure 1b.1.7. MR images of a simple bone cyst located in the left mandible of a 15-year-old female patient. The axial MR images show homogeneous iso-intensity on T1WI (left) and homogeneous marked hyperintensity with clear borders on T2WI (center). The contrast-enhanced T1WI acquired approximately 6 min after the administration of contrast agent (right) shows marked enhancement of the margin and slight enhancement of the inner part of the cyst cavity.

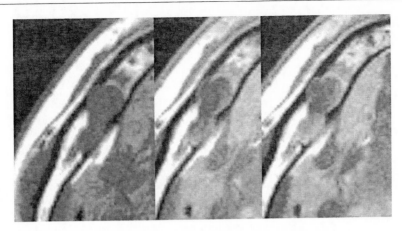

Figure 1b.1.8. MR images of a simple bone cyst located in the right mandible of a 25-year-old female patient. The axial MR images show homogeneous isointensity with clear borders on T1WI (left). The contrast-enhanced T1WI acquired approximately 480 seconds (center) and 1000 seconds (right) after the administration of contrast agent show slight enhancement of the inner part of the cyst cavity. The signal intensity of the inner part of the cyst cavity increased over time.

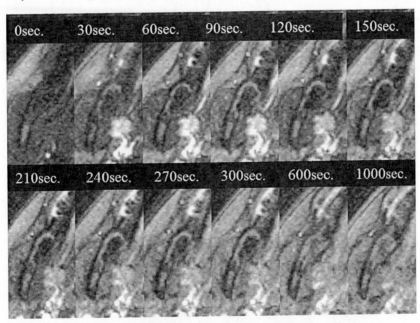

Figure 1b.1.9. Dynamic contrast-enhanced MR images of a simple bone cyst located in the right mandible of a 40-year-old female patient (Selected images. The time indicated on the figure represents the time that had elapsed since the administration of contrast agent.) This series of dynamic contrast-enhanced MR images clearly shows the gradual spreading of contrast enhancement from the margin to the inner part of the cyst cavity. Adapted from reference no.3 (Yanagi Y et al. Usefulness of MRI and dynamic contrast-enhanced MRI for differential diagnosis of simple bone cysts from true cysts in the jaw. Oral Surg Oral Med Oral Pathol Oral Radiol Endod. 2010;110:364–9. doi:10.1016/j.tripleo.2010.05.001.)

Many investigators believe that the cavities of simple bone cysts are "empty". However, this finding has only been seen during surgical procedures. On the other hand, the cavity displays fluid-like density on CT [6] and fluid-like signal intensity on MR images [2-5]. No previously reported cases have displayed an air-like density on CT or air-like signals within the lesion on MRI.

References

[1]   Barnes L, Evenson JW, Reichart P, Sidransky D, editors. World Health Organization classification of tumours. *Pathology and genetics of head and neck tumours.* Lyon: IARC Press; 2007.

[2]   Matsuzaki h, Asaumi j, Yanagi Y, Konouchi H, Honda Y, Hisatomi M, Shigehara H, Kishi K. MR imaging in the assessment of a solitary bone cyst. *Eur J Radiol Extra.* 2003;45:37-42.

[3]   Yanagi Y, Asaumi J, Unetsubo T, Ashida M, Takenobu T, Hisatomi M, Matsuzaki H, Konouchi H, Katase N, Nagatsuka H. Usefulness of MRI and dynamic contrast-enhanced MRI for differential diagnosis of simple bone cysts from true cysts in the jaw. *Oral Surg Oral Med Oral Pathol Oral Radiol Endod.* 2010;110:364–9. doi:10.1016/j.tripleo.2010.05.001.

[4]   Tanaka H, Westesson P-L, Emmings FG, Harashi AH. Simple bone cyst of the mandibular condyle: report of a case. *J Oral Maxillofac Surg* 1996;54:1454-8.

[5]   Ogasawara T, Kitagawa Y, Ogawa T, Yamada T, Yamamoto S, Hayashi K. Simple bone cyst of the mandibular condyle with sever osteoarthritis: report of a case. *J Oral Pathol Med* 1999;28:377-80.

[6]   Suei Y, Taguchi A, Kurabayashi T, Kobayashi F, Nojiri M, Tanimoto K. Simple bone cyst: investigation on the presence of gas in the cavity using computed tomography. *Oral Surg Oral Med Oral Pathol* 1998;86:592-4.

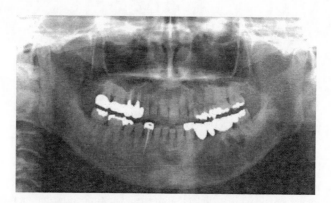

Figure 1b.2.1. An aneurysmal bone cyst in a 39-year-old female patient. A panoramic radiograph detected a large expansile, multilocular lesion with a thin bony rim in the left mandible, which extended from the left first premolar to the mandibular ramus. Adapted from reference no.5 (Wakasa T et al. Aneurysmal bone cyst of the mandible: a report of 2 cases and a review of the literature. Jpn J Oral Diagn/Oral Med. 2002;15:352–8).

1b.2. Aneurysmal Bone Cyst

Aneurysmal bone cyst (ABC) is a relatively rare, benign bone lesion. The WHO classifies ABC as a bone-related lesion and defines it as 'an expansile osteolytic lesion, which is often multilocular, with blood filled spaces separated by fibrous septa containing osteoclast type giant cells and reactive bone' [1]. Aneurysmal bone cysts are commonly found on the metaphyses of the long bones of the extremities. Jawbone involvement is also rare and mostly occurs in the posterior mandible. Aneurysmal bone cysts usually occur in the first two decades of life, and most studies have found a slightly increased incidence in women. Although the etiology of this lesion is unknown, aneurysmal bone cysts occur as primary or secondary tumors. Although aneurysmal bone cysts are locally aggressive, they are thought to be caused by a reactive process following a fracture or to be associated with benign conditions such as giant cell tumor, chondroblastoma, chondromyxoid fibroma, and fibrous dysplasia. However, they can also arise de novo, and some recent molecular genetic studies have suggested that some aneurysmal bone cysts develop via a neoplastic process [2]. More recently, metastasis of primary aneurysmal bone cyst was reported in the literature [3].

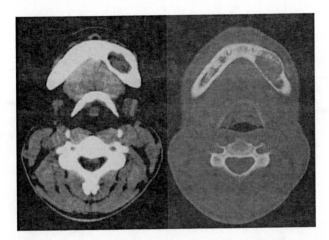

Figure 1b.2.2. CT images of the same patient as shown in Figure 1b.2.1. Axial CT images showing buccolingual bony expansion and cortical thinning. The lesion displays low attenuation values of between 20 and 30 Hounsfield units, which are consistent with a liquid-like density.

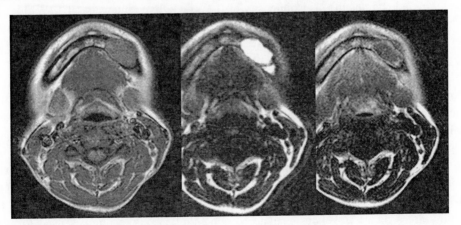

Figure 1b.2.3. Axial MR images of the same patient as shown in Figure 1b.2.1. (a) T1WI (left) showing almost homogeneous isointensity. (b) Fat suppressed T2WI MR image (center) showing homogeneous marked hyperintensity. (c) Fat suppressed contrast-enhanced T1WI MR image (right) showing slight hyperintensity at the periphery of the lesion. The center of the lesion displays weak contrast enhancement. Adapted from reference no.5 (Wakasa T, et al. Aneurysmal bone cyst of the mandible: a report of 2 cases and a review of the literature. Jpn J Oral Diagn/Oral Med. 2002;15:352–8).

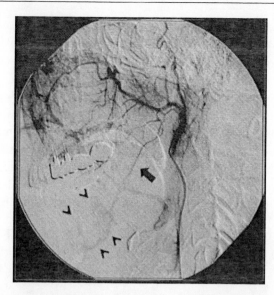

Figure 1b.2.4. Digital subtraction angiography. The lesion was supplied by the left inferior alveolar artery (arrow). The tumor blush effect was relatively weak (arrowhead), and no arteriovenous shunt was depicted. Adapted from reference no.6 (Yanagi Y et al. The utility of three-dimensional dynamic contrast-enhanced magnetic resonance imaging in delineating vessel-rich regions: a case report of an aneurysmal bone cyst of the mandible. Oral Radiology 2010;26:110-5, DOI 10.1007/s11282-010-0048-3).

Radiographically, aneurysmal bone cysts appear as a well-defined, uniloculated, or multiloculated osteolytic lesion combined with expansion of the cortical bone. Perforation and/or destruction of the cortical bone are also often observed (Figure 1b.2.1). These findings are easily delineated by CT, which sometimes also detects the fluid-fluid level sign (Figure 1b.2.2). MRI can reveal the detailed internal structures of the lesion, including the fluid–fluid level sign, hemorrhaging, and internal septa. The MR features of aneurysmal bone cysts generally include homogeneous isointensity on T1WI and hyperintensity on T2WI [4, 5]. The internal parts of the blood-pooling cavity usually display hyper- to marked hyperintensity on T2WI but their signal intensity can vary according to the degree of hemorrhaging. In addition, the signal intensities of areas of blood flow vary according to the flow rate. For the same reason, the contrast enhancement of areas of blood flow also varies (Figure 1b.2.3) [6].

Angiography is sometimes recommended as a means of preoperatively evaluating intralesional blood flow in order to avoid unexpected bleeding during surgery. Intra-arterial digital subtraction angiography (DSA) is currently the reference standard for diagnostic angiography but does carry some risks (Figure 1b.2.4). Although CT angiography is less invasive than catheter angiography, the use of iodinated contrast medium poses a risk of contrast-induced nephropathy [7]. Where possible, the vascularity of the lesion should be evaluated using non-invasive methods because aneurysmal bone cysts do not always have high flow areas or arteriovenous fistulae. Among the various techniques used to evaluate blood flow, the use of MRI with Gadolinium-based contrast agents is relatively safe considering the low risk of complications (Figure 1b.2.5) [6].

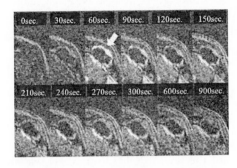

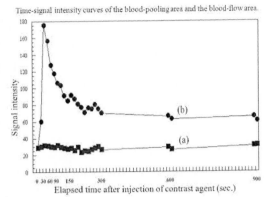

Figure 1b.2.5. Dynamic contrast-enhanced MR images (left) and time-signal intensity curves of the blood-pooling area and the areas of blood flow (right) in the same lesion as shown in Figure 1b.2.1. (Selected images. The time indicated on the figure represents the time that had elapsed after the administration of contrast agent.). Marked enhancement was observed at the periphery of the buccal side of the lesion during the early phase after contract agent injection (arrow). The signal intensity of this area showed a rapid increase in the early phase after contract agent injection, followed by a rapid decrease until 150 seconds. No contrast enhancement was observed in the center of the cyst cavity. The area that displayed rapid enhancement had blood flowing through it, and the center of the cyst cavity was thought to be the blood-pooling area, which did not have blood flowing through it. The time-signal intensity curve of the blood-pooling area did not show any change in signal intensity until approximately 900 seconds after the administration of contrast agent (a). The time-signal intensity curve of the blood-flow area showed a rapid increase in SI during the early phase after contract agent injection, followed by a rapid decrease until 150 seconds and a gradual decrease until approximately 900 seconds after the administration of Gd-DTPA (b). Adapted from reference no.6 (Yanagi Y et al. The utility of three-dimensional dynamic contrast-enhanced magnetic resonance imaging in delineating vessel-rich regions: a case report of an aneurysmal bone cyst of the mandible. Oral Radiology 2010;26:110-5, DOI 10.1007/s11282-010-0048-3).

References

[1]   Barnes L, Evenson JW, Reichart P, Sidransky D, editors. World Health Organization classification of tumours. Pathology and genetics of head and neck tumours. Lyon: IARC Press; 2005.

[2]   Unni KK, Inwards C, Mayo *Foundation for Medical Education and Research.* Dahlin's bone tumors : general aspects and data on 10,165 cases, 6th ed. Philadelphia: Lippincott Williams & Wilkins; 2010.

[3]   van de Luijtgaarden, A. C., Veth, R. P., Slootweg, P. J., Wijers-Koster, P. M., Schultze Kool, L. J., Bovee, J. V., van der Graaf, W. T. Metastatic potential of an aneurysmal bone cyst. *Virchows Arch.* 2009; 455: 455–459

[4]   Asaumi J, Konouchi H, Hisatomi M, Matsuzaki H, Shigehara H, Honda Y, Kishi K. MR features of aneurysmal bone cyst of the mandible and characteristics distinguishing it from other lesions. *Eur J Radiol.* 2003;45:108-12.

[5]   Wakasa T, Asaumi JI, Konouchi H, Honda Y, Kishi K. Aneurysmal bone cyst of the mandible: a report of 2 cases and a review of the literature. *Jpn J Oral Diagn/Oral Med.* 2002;15:352–8.

[6]   Yanagi Y, Fujita M, Hisatomi M, Matsuzaki H, Konouchi H, Katase N, Nagatsuka H, Asaumi J. The utility of three-dimensional dynamic contrast-enhanced magnetic resonance imaging in delineating vessel-rich regions: a case report of an aneurysmal bone cyst of the mandible. *Oral Radiology* 2010;26:110-5

[7]   Walsh SR, Tang T, Gaunt ME, Boyle JR. Contrast-induced nephropathy. *J Endovasc Ther.* 2007;14:92-100.

1b.3. Static Bone Cavity

Static bone cavity is classified as a pseudocyst of the jaw. In 1942, Stafne [1] was the first to report a series of asymptomatic radiolucent "bone cavities" in the angle of the mandible. Several synonyms have been given to these lesions: static bone cavity, idiopathic bone cavity [2], static bone cyst [3], and mandibular embryonic defect [4]. The incidence of static bone cavity ranges from 0.1 to 1.28% [5-7]. No treatment is required for static bone cavity as it has an excellent prognosis. Generally, static bone cavities are located beneath the root apex and alveolar canal, and this characteristic location is considered to be a diagnostic radiological feature of static bone cavity. Most cases exhibit well-defined areas of radiolucency with dense radiopaque borders. The bone defect always opens on the lingual cortical margin [8], and the size of the lesion ranges from 0.5 to 2 cm. As the size of the defect rarely changes, they are considered to be static lesions. Therefore, it is important to evaluate the contents of static bone cavities in order to obtain a definitive diagnosis. It has been reported that static bone cavities contain salivary glands, fat tissue, soft tissue, and vascular structures [9-12]. The etiology of static bone cavities has still not been fully elucidated [13-19]. However, some studies have suggested that the entrapment of the salivary gland parenchyma in the mandible during mandibular development is one possible cause [13-15, 20].

Sialography has been suggested to be useful for diagnosing static bone cavities. Whilst sialography might be useful for diagnosing lesions containing salivary gland tissue [21], it is not suggested to be a suitable diagnostic modality for assessing invasiveness. CT is non-invasive, easy to perform, and highly recommended for both diagnosis and follow-up [8]. MRI is also proposed to be a useful non-invasive diagnostic tool for static bone cavities [9]. Since MRI is able to clearly visualize the characteristics of soft tissue lesions, it is ideal for identifying the contents of static bone cavities. Static bone cavities are usually discovered during dental examinations, and they can easily be differentiated from mandibular cysts. However, static bone cavities rarely develop in the anterior mandible. For example, in a review of 310 static bone cavity cases Philpsen *et al.* [22] found that only 40 were located anteriorly; thus, the anterior variant of static bone cavity might be difficult for dental clinicians to diagnose [23]. As for the differential diagnoses of static bone cavity, radicular cyst, residual cyst, and odontogenic cyst are the most frequent diagnoses. In the anterior mandible, it has been suggested that static bone cavities are associated with the sublingual gland or aberrant salivary gland tissue [5, 6, 24, 25]. In particular, MRI has been shown to be helpful for identifying unusually anteriorly located cases [26]. Using MRI, Bornstein et al. demonstrated that static bone cavities in the mandibular canine-premolar region contained salivary gland tissue [26].

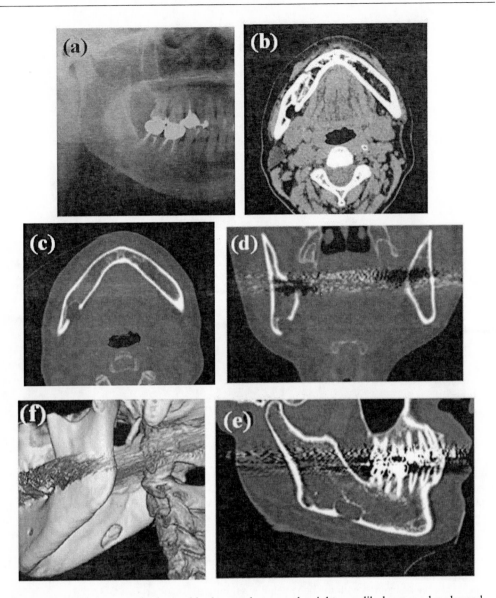

Figure 1b.3.1. A static bone cavity located in the area between the right mandibular second molar and the mandibular angle in a 61-year-old female. (a) Panoramic tomography revealed a 2x1.5 cm bone defect located in the area between the mandibular second molar and the mandibular angle. Radiographically, it was observed as a well-defined, unilocular, ovoid radiolucent area. A thin but dense radiopaque border surrounded the defect. The radiolucent area was located inferior to the mandibular canal, and its mandibular inferior border was intact. (b) An axial CT scan revealed a focal concavity of cortical bone on the lingual surface of the mandible. On axial CT images obtained with the soft tissue window setting, the CT number of the static bone cavity contents was -100 HU, which was indicative of adipose tissue. The attenuation of the soft tissue was different from that of the submandibular gland tissue. (c) Axial CT images obtained with the bone window setting. (d) A coronal CT image obtained with the bone window setting. (e) A sagittal CT image obtained with the bone window setting. (f) Reconstructed 3D-CT.

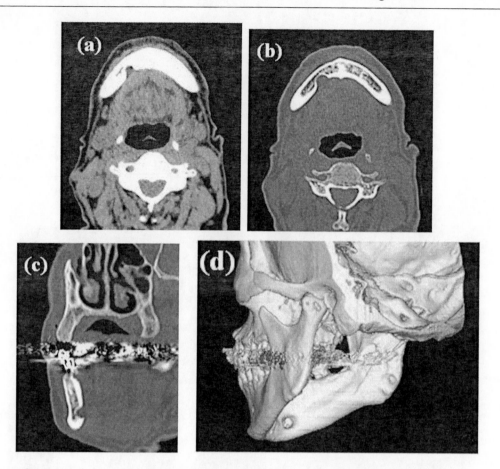

Figure1b.3.2.A static bone cavity in the anterior mandible of a 78-year-old male. (a). An axial CT image obtained with the soft tissue window setting. A 2x2 cm area of radiolucency was detected in the lingual canine region of the right mandible. The lingual cortical bone and mandibular inferior border were intact. An axial CT examination performed with the soft tissue window setting revealed that the contents of the static bone cavity had a similar iso-CT number to the surrounding soft tissue (a). Thus, the static bone cavity might have been filled with portions of sublingual salivary gland tissue rather than adipose tissue. Static bone cavities in the anterior mandible are relatively rare, but dentists should be aware of their existence. (b) An axial CT image obtained with the bone window setting. (c) A coronal CT image obtained with the bone window setting. (d) Reconstructed 3D-CT.

References

[1]   Stafne EC. Bone cavities situated near the angle of the mandible. *J Am Dent Assoc* 1942;29:1969-72.

[2]   Stevens ME. Idiopathic bone cavity of mandible. *Bull Tri Cty Dent Soc* 1965;15(2):7.

[3]   Neely AR, Ruhlman CD. Roentgeno-oddities. Static bone cyst. *Oral Surg Oral Med Oral Pathol* 1966;22(6):751.

[4]   Jacobs MH. The traumatic bone cysts. *Oral Surg Oral Med Oral Pathol* 1955;8(9):940-9.

[5]   Buchner A, Carpenter WM, Merrell PW, Leider AS. Anterior lingual mandibular salivary gland defect. Evaluation of twenty-four cases. *Oral Surg Oral Med Oral Pathol* 1991;71: 131-6.

[6]   Apruzzese D, Longoni S. Stafne cyst in an anterior location. *J Oral Maxillofac Surg* 1999;57: 333-8.

[7]   Oikarinen VJ, Julku M. An orthopanthomographic study of developmental bone defects (Stafne's idiopathic bone cavities). *Int J Oral Surg* 1974;3:71-6.

[8]   Slasky BS, Bar-Ziv J. Lingual mandibular bony defects: CT in the buccolingual plane. *J Comput Assist Tomogr* 1996;20:439-43.

[9]   Branstetter BF, Weissman JL, Kaplan SB. Imaging of a Stafne bone cavity: what MR adds and why a new name is needed. *Am J Neuroradiol* 1999;20:587-9.

[10] Ariji E, Fujiwara N, Tabata O, Nakayama E, Kanda S, Shiratsuchi Y, Oka M. Stafne's bone cavity. Classification based on outline and content determined by computed tomography. *Oral Surg Oral Med Oral Pathol* 1993;76:375-80.

[11] Minowa K, Inoue N, Sawamura T, Matsuda A, Totsuka T, Nakamura M. Evaluation of static bone cavities with CT and MRI. *Dentomaxillofac Radiol* 2003;32:2-7.

[12] Damante JH, Camarini ET, Silver MA. Lingual mandibular bone defect: a developmental entity. *Dentomaxillofac Radiol* 1998;27:58.

[13] Amaral WJ, Jacobs DS. Aberrant salivary gland defect in the mandible: report of a case. *Oral Surg Oral Med Oral Pathol* 1961;14:748-52.

[14] Hayes H. Aberrant submaxillary gland tissue presenting as a cyst of the jaw: report of a case. *Oral Surg Oral Med Oral Pathol* 1961;14:313-6.

[15] Choukas NC. Developmental submandibular gland defect of the mandible. Review of the literature and report of two cases. *J Oral Surg* 1973;31:209-11.

[16] Shimizu M, Osa N, Okumura K, Yoshiura K. CT analysis of the static bone defects of the mandible. *Dentomaxillofac Radiol* 2006;35:95-102.

[17] Minowa K, Inoue N, Izumiyama Y, Ashikaga Y, Chu B, Maravilla KR, Totsuka Y, Nakamura M. Static bone cavity of the mandible: computed tomography findings with histopathologic correlation. *Acta Radiol* 2006;47:706-9.

[18] Neville BW, Damm DD, Allen CM, Bouquot JB. *Oral and maxillofacial pathology.* 2nd edn. Philadelphia: Saunders, 2002:23-4.

[19] Glenn EL, Miro M. Stafne's mandibular lingual cortical defect. *J Maxillofac Surg* 1985;13:172-6.

[20] Tolman DE, Stafne EC. Developmental bone defects of the mandible. *Oral Surg Oral Med Oral Pathol* 1967;24(4):488-90.

[21] Oikarinen VJ, Wolf J, Julku M. A stereosialographic study of developmental mandibular bone defects (Stafne's idiopathic bone cavities). *Int J Oral Surg* 1975;4:51-4.

[22] Philipsen HP, Takata T, Reichart PA, Sato S, Suei Y. Lingual and buccal mandibular bone depressions: a review based on 583 cases from a world-wide literature survey, including 69 new cases from Japan. *Dentomaxillofac Radiol* 2002;31:281-90.

[23] Barak S, Katz J, Mintz S. Anterior lingual mandibular salivary gland defect—a dilemma in diagnosis. *Br J Oral Maxillofac Surg* 1993; 31: 318-20.

[24] Miller AS, Winnick M. Salivary gland inclusion in the anterior mandible. Report of a case with a review of the literature on aberrant salivary gland tissue and neoplasms. *Oral Surg Oral Med Oral Pathol* 1971;31(6):790-7.

[25] Tominaga K, Kuga Y, Kubota K, Ohba T. Stafne's bone cavity in the anterior mandible: report of a case. *Dentomaxillofac Radiol* 1990; 19(1):28-30.

[26] Borns tein MM, Wiest R, Balsiger R, Reichart PA. Anterior Stafne's bone cavity mimicking a periapical lesion of endodontic origin: report of two cases. *J Endod* 2009;35(11):1598-602.

2. CYSTS THAT AFFECT SOFT TISSUE

2.1. Nasolabial Cyst

Nasolabial cysts are unilateral (rarely bilateral) soft tissue lesions that occur adjacent to the alveolar process near the base of the nostril. Nasolabial cysts are thought to be remnants of the embryonic nasolacrimal duct or the lower anterior portion of the mature duct. Nasolabial cysts are often lined by a stratified squamous, cuboidal, or respiratory epithelium. The lining is surrounded by a cystic wall composed of fibrous connective tissue, abundant collagen I fibers, and numerous inflammatory cells in the subepithelial region and might also contain cartilage and accessory salivary gland elements [1]. This cyst does not arise within the bone, but can cause superficial erosion of the outer surface of the maxilla.

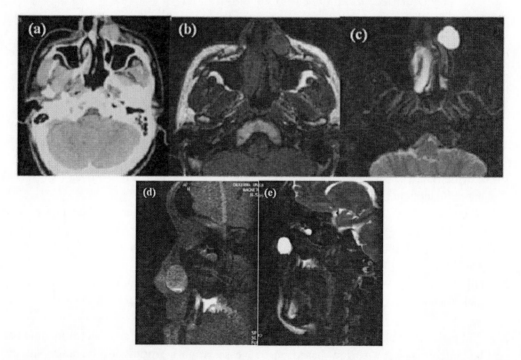

Figure 2.1.1. A nasolabial cyst in a 30-year-old male. Axial CT images (a) obtained using the soft tissue window show a well-defined soft tissue mass in the left nasolabial fold that displayed homogeneous soft tissue radiodensity and bone structure preservation. Axial (T1WI: b and T2WI: c) and sagittal (T1WI: d and T2WI: e) MR images displayed homogeneous isointensity on T1WI and hyperintensity on T2WI. This indicates that the interior of the lesion included a fluid component. The lesion was diagnosed as a nasolabial cyst on the basis of its MR features and location.

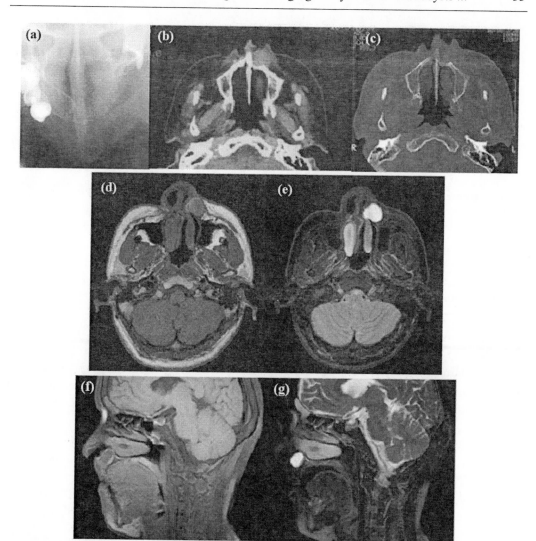

Figure 2.1.2. A nasolabial cyst in a 67-year-old female. An occlusal radiograph (a) did not show any of the lesion's features. Axial CT images obtained with the soft tissue window (b) and bone window (c) settings showed superficial erosion of the outer surface of the maxilla. Axial (T1WI: d and T2WI: e) and sagittal (T1WI: f and T2WI: g) MR images revealed a well-defined area of homogeneous hypointensity on T1WI and hyperintensity on T2WI as well as the two dimensional extent of the lesion. This indicates that the interior of the lesion included a fluid component. The lesion was diagnosed as a nasolabial cyst on the basis of its imaging features and location. It was also possible to clearly visualize the extent of the lesion.

Conventional radiographs can not visualize the features of nasolabial cysts except in cases in which they cause significant maxillary bone erosion because the cysts consist of fluid surrounded by a cyst wall. Thus, radiographically, nasolabial cysts might not be recognized unless they are examined in the presence of radiopaque material. CT and MRI can clearly depict the contents and margins of nasolabial cysts. CT images of nasolabial cysts display a well-demarcated low- to high-density cystic lesion lateral to the pyriform aperture. The SI variation is presumably caused by the different viscosities of the intracystic fluid [2, 3]. Occasionally, adjacent bony erosion of the anterior maxillary buccal cortex occurs, probably as a result of cystic pressure (Figure 2.1.2b, c) [3, 4]. Such adjacent bony erosion can be seen on CT and MRI. The MRI features of nasolabial cysts include low to isointensity on T1WI and hyperintensity on T2WI (Figure 2.1.1, 2). MR images of nasolabial cysts show various signal intensities, especially on T1WI, due to their different serous to mucinous contents and variations in the protein content of their intracystic fluid. On contrast-enhanced MR images [5-8], the cyst wall is enhanced, but its inner contents are not. Nasolabial cysts can be diagnosed according to the location and features of the lesion, especially if the lesion is accompanied by adjacent bony erosion and a liquid-like interior.

References

[1]   Kramer IRH, Pindborg JJ, Shear M. *Histological typing of odontogenic tumours,* 2nd ed. New York: Springer, 1992.

[2]   Marcoviceanu MP, Metzger MC, Deppe H, Freudenberg N, Kassem A, Pautke C, Hohlweg-Majert B. Report of rare bilateral nasolabial cysts. *J Craniomaxillofac Surg* 2009;37(2):83-6.

[3]   Sazgar AA, Sadeghi M, Yazdi AK, Ojani L.Transnasal endoscopic marsupialization of bilateral nasoalveolar cysts. *Int J Oral Maxillofac Surg* 2009;38(11):1210-1.

[4]   Kato H, Kanematsu M, Kusunoki Y, Shibata T, Murakami H, Mizuta K, Ito Y, Hirose Y. Nasoalveolar cyst: imaging findings in three cases.*Clin Imaging* 2007;31(3):206-9.

[5]   Tanimoto K, Kakimoto N, Nishiyama H, Murakami S, Kishino M. MRI of nasoalveolar cyst: case report. *Oral Surg Oral Med Oral Pathol Oral Radiol Endod* 2005;99(2):221-4.

[6]   Sumer AP, Celenk P, Sumer M, Telcioglu NT, Gunhan O. Nasolabial cyst: case report with CT and MRI findings. *Oral Surg Oral Med Oral Pathol Oral Radiol Endod* 2010;109(2):e92-4.

[7]   Aquilino RN, Bazzo VJ, Faria RJ, Eid NL, Bóscolo FN. Nasolabial cyst: presentation of a clinical case with CT and MR images. *Braz J Otorhinolaryngol* 2008;74(3):467-71.

[8]   Curé JK, Osguthorpe JD, Van Tassel P. MR of nasolabial cysts. *AJNR Am J Neuroradiol* 1996;17(3):585-8.

2.2. Mucous Retention Cyst

Mucous retention cyst is a common, benign, mucus-containing cystic lesion of the minor salivary glands in the oral cavity. Some authors prefer the term mucocele since most of these lesions are not true cysts as they lack an epithelial lining. Mucous retention cysts can be located directly under the mucosa (superficial mucocele), in the upper submucosa (classic mucocele), or in the lower corium (deep mucocele) and are categorized into two types according to the histological features of their cyst walls: mucous extravasation cysts, which are composed of mucous pools surrounded by granulation tissue (92%), and mucous retention cysts, which have an epithelial lining (8%) [1]. Mucous cysts develop in various oral and maxillofacial membranes such as the lips, buccal membrane, the tongue, the floor of the mouth (including ranulas), and the maxillary sinus [2-7]. CT scans frequently demonstrate a well-defined mass with a density similar to that of water. MRI depict a lesion that displays homogeneous hypointensity on T1WI, whereas T2WI reveal a lesion that demonstrates hyperintensity and sharp borders. On contrast-enhanced T1WI, the inner part of the lesion does not show any enhancement (Figure 2.2.1, 2).

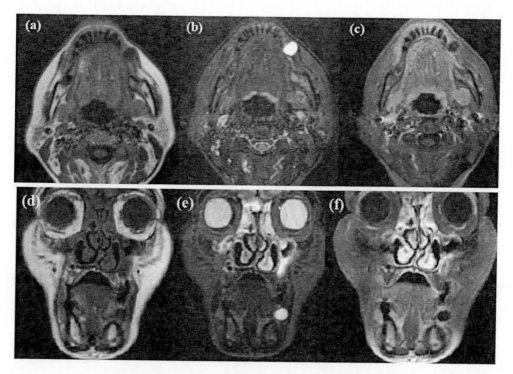

Figure 2.2.1. A mucous retention cyst in the buccal membrane of a 19-year-old male. Both axial (upper) and coronal (lower) MRI show hypointensity on T1WI (a, d), hyperintensity on T2WI (c, f), and no enhancement of the inner part of the lesion on contrast enhanced T1WI (b, e). These MR features indicate that the lesion contained simple fluid and that the contrast agent had not entered its interior. Thus, the lesion was considered to be a true fluid-containing cyst with a cystic wall. The lesion was diagnosed as a mucocele on the basis of its MR features and location.

Mucous cysts can be diagnosed relatively easily according to their location and MRI features, especially if they include simple fluid.

References

[1]   Kramer IRH, Pindborg JJ, Shear M. *Histological typing of odontogenic tumours, 2nd ed.* New York: Springer, 1992.

[2]   Wu CW, Kao YH, Chen CM, Hsu HJ, Chen CM, Huang IY. Mucoceles of the oral cavity in pediatric patients. *Kaohsiung J Med Sci* 2011;27(7):276-9.

[3]   Pedron IG, Galletta VC, Azevedo LH, Corrêa L. Treatment of mucocele of the lower lip with diode laser in pediatric patients: presentation of 2 clinical cases. *Pediatr Dent* 2010;32(7):539-41.

[4]   Tilaveridis I, Lazaridou M, Lazaridis N. The use of magnification and microsurgical instruments for the excision of lower lip mucoceles. *J Oral Maxillofac Surg* 2011;69(5):1408-10.

[5]   Adachi P, Soubhia AM, Horikawa FK, Shinohara EH. Mucocele of the glands of Blandin-Nuhn--clinical, pathological, and therapeutical aspects. *Oral Maxillofac Surg* 2011;15(1):11-3.

[6]   Marques J, Figueiredo R, Aguirre-Urizar JM, Berini-Aytés L, Gay-Escoda C. Root resorption caused by a maxillary sinus mucocele: a case report. *Oral Surg Oral Med Oral Pathol Oral Radiol Endod* 2011;111(5):e37-40.

[7]   Chi AC, Lambert PR 3rd, Richardson MS, Neville BW. Oral mucoceles: a clinicopathologic review of 1,824 cases, including unusual variants. *J Oral Maxillofac Surg* 2011;69(4):1086-93.

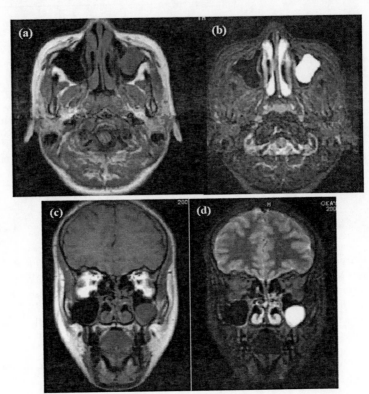

Figure 2.2.2. A mucocele in the left maxillary sinus of a 13-year-old female. Both axial (upper) and coronal (lower) MRI displayed hypointensity on T1WI (a, c) and hyperintensity on T2WI (b, d), indicating that the lesion contained simple fluid. The lesion was diagnosed as a mucocele on the basis of its MR features and location.

2.3. Dermoid/epidermoid Cyst

Dermoid and epidermoid cysts are developmental cystic malformations. There are two theories to explain their embryogenesis. In the first theory, dermoid and epidermoid cysts originate from embryonic cells of the first and second branchial arches, which fuse during the third and fourth weeks in utero. The second theory suggests that these cysts occur when the ectodermal surface fails to completely separate from the underlying neural tube.

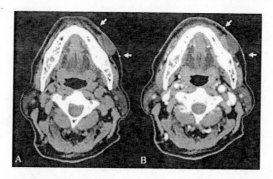

Figure 2.3.1. CT images of an epidermoid cyst in the left buccal region of a 74-year-old male. An axial CT image shows an oval mass in the left subcutaneous buccal region that displays homogeneous hypodensity (A). On a CE-CT image (B), neither the central zone of the lesion nor its cyst wall show any enhancement. The arrows indicate wire markers.

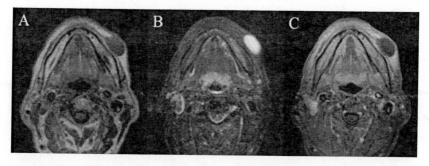

Figure 2.3.2. MR images of an epidermoid cyst in the left buccal region of a 74-year-old male. Axial MR images of an epidermoid cyst in the left buccal region showing a cystic mass that displayed almost homogeneous isointensity on T1WI (A) and slightly heterogeneous iso- to hyperintensity on STIR images (B). Neither the central nor peripheral zone of the cystic mass displayed any enhancement on axial CE-T1WI (C).

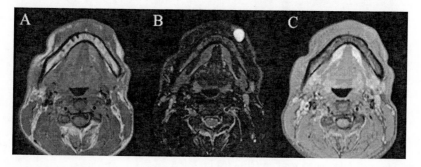

Figure 2.3.3. MR images of an epidermoid cyst in the left lower lip of a 28-year-old male. The epidermoid cyst in the left lower lip appeared as a round mass with a well-defined margin, which showed slightly heterogeneous hypo- to isointensity on axial T1WI (A) and iso- to hyperintensity on axial STIR images (B). The central zone of the lesion did not show any enhancement, whereas the peripheral zone displayed rim enhancement on axial CE-T1WI (C).

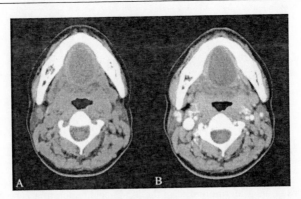

Figure 2.3.4. CT images of a dermoid cyst in the floor of the mouth of a 40-year-old female. A large mass, which displayed homogenous hypodensity on axial CT images (A), was located on the midline of the floor of the mouth. (B) On a CE-CT image, the central zone of the lesion did not show any enhancement, whereas the peripheral zone showed slight thin rim enhancement.

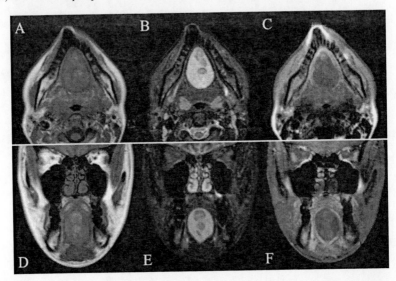

Figure 2.3.5. MR images of a dermoid cyst of the floor of the mouth in a 40-year-old female. A large oval mass on the floor of the mouth was found to be a cystic lesion with a well-defined margin. The lesion included some regions (dermal appendages) that displayed different signal intensities from the liquid component on coronal and sagittal MR images (A, B, D, E). On T1WI (A, D), the liquid component of the lesion displayed almost homogeneous slightly isointensity and dermal appendages that demonstrated heterogeneous iso- to hyperintensity. On T2WI (B, E), the former lesion displayed heterogeneous hyperintensity and the latter showed heterogeneous isointensity. Only the peripheral zone; i.e., the cyst wall, was enhanced on CE-T1WI (C, F).

The incidence of dermoid and epidermoid cysts is reported to be approximately 7% in the head and neck region [1]. In contrast, dermoid and epidermoid cysts account for less than 0.01% of all oral cysts, and most dermoid and epidermoid cysts in the oral region affect the floor of the mouth [2-5].

Histopathologically, dermoid cysts are lined by a keratinizing squamous epithelium and contain fat, hair follicles, or other skin appendages in their cyst walls. On the other hand, epidermoid cysts are lined by a keratinizing squamous epithelium without dermal appendages. These differences in the histopathological findings of epidermoid and dermoid cysts have a perceptible influence on their imaging diagnosis.

CT and MRI are useful modalities for diagnosing dermoid and epidermoid cysts as they arise from soft tissues. On CT, epidermoid cysts commonly appear as an oval mass that displays homogenous hypodensity compared with that of the surrounding muscles (Figure 2.3.1), and its MRI features include a unilocular cystic mass displaying fluid retention; i.e., that appears iso- to hyperintense on T1WI and hyperintense on T2WI (or STIR images) (Figure 2.3.2, 3). This MRI finding of epidermoid cysts is not unique; therefore, epidermoid cysts are often indistinguishable from other soft tissue cystic lesions (e.g., thyroglossal cyst, ranula, branchial cleft cyst, etc.) depending on their localization. On the other hand, dermoid cysts display characteristic findings on CT and MRI due to the presence of dermal appendages in their cyst cavities. The CT images of this lesion sometimes include areas of calcification in the inner part of the lesion (Figure 2.3.4) [6]. MRI of dermoid cysts display a unique cystic mass containing dermal appendages, which show various signal intensities, in the cyst cavity (Figure 2.3.5). Therefore, dermoid cysts are relatively easy to distinguish on MRI, unlike epidermoid cysts.

References

[1]   New GB, Erich JB. Dermoid cysts of the head and neck. *Surg Gynecol Obstet* 1937;65:48-55.
[2]   Brown CA, Baker RD. Dermoid cyst: report of case. *J Oral Surg* 1972;30:55-8.
[3]   Seward GR. Dermoid cysts of the floor of the mouth. Br J Oral Surg 1965;3:36-47.
[4]   Howell CJ. The sublingual dermoid cyst. Report of five cases and review of the literature. *Oral Surg Oral Med Oral Pathol* 1985;59:578-80.
[5]   Rapidis AD, Angelopoulos AP, Scouteris C. Dermoid cyst of the floor of the mouth. *Report of a case. Br J Oral Surg* 1981;19:43-51.
[6]   Wong KT, Lee YY, King AD, Ahuja AT. Imaging of cystic or cyst-like neck masses. *Clin Radiol* 2008;63:613-22.

2.4. Epidermal Cyst

Epidermal cyst is the most common type of skin cyst and is also known as epidermal inclusion cyst, sebaceous cyst, or infundibular cyst. They can occur anywhere on the body but tend to occur on the face, neck, and trunk. Epidermal cysts can occur at any age, although they most commonly arise in the third or fourth decade of life. True epidermal inclusion cysts result from the implantation of epithelial elements in the dermis. The implanted tissue can become cystic and filled with laminated keratin, cholesterol crystals, and debris. Most lesions arise from the follicular infundibulum; therefore, this lesion is more generally known as epidermoid cyst. The primary symptom of this lesion is a painless nodule or pale lump affecting the skin. Epidermal cysts are generally pale colored and are movable under the skin. Histopathologically, epidermal cysts are filled with keratin debris and lined by a wall composed of a stratified squamous epithelium.

On CT, epidermal cysts appear as an oval mass that is located immediately below the skin and displays almost homogenous hypo- to isodensity compared with that of the muscles. When an epidermal cyst becomes infected, the surrounding fatty layer of the mass displays hyperdensity. On MRI, epidermal cysts commonly appear as a mass that displays homogenous hypointensity on T1WI and hyperintensity on T2WI (STIR images). However, some epidermal cysts contain keratin debris. In these cases, MR images display heterogeneous signal intensity [1-3]. The differential diagnoses of this lesion include branchial cleft cyst, dermoid cyst, calcinosis cutis lipoma, and milium.

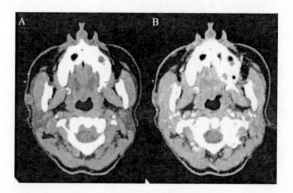

Figure 2.4.1. CT images of an epidermal cyst in the right buccal region of a 60-year-old female. An axial CT image showed an oval mass in the right subcutaneous buccal region that displayed almost homogeneous isodensity (A). On a CE-CT image (B), neither the central zone of the lesion nor the cyst wall showed any enhancement.

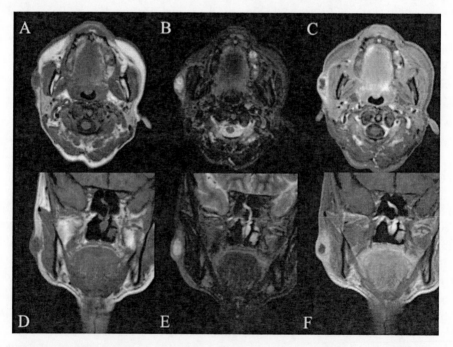

Figure 2.4.2. . MR images of an epidermal cyst in the right buccal region of a 60-year-old female. An oval mass in the right subcutaneous buccal region displayed heterogeneous hypo- to isointensity on coronal and sagittal T1WI (A, D) and heterogeneous iso- to hyperintensity on coronal and sagittal STIR images (A, D). On CE-T1WI (C, F), the peripheral zone of the lesion displayed marked enhancement.

References

[1]   Sundaram M, McGuire MH, Herbold DR, Beshany SE, Fletcher JW. High signal intensity soft tissue masses on T1 weighted pulsing sequences. *Skeletal Radiol* 1987;16(1):30-6.

[2]   Shibata T, Hatori M, Satoh T, Ehara S, Kokubun S. Magnetic resonance imaging features of epidermoid cyst in the extremities. *Arch Orthop Trauma Surg* 2003;123(5):239-41.

[3]   Kransdorf MJ, Jelinek JS, Moser RP, Jr., Utz JA, Brower AC, Hudson TM, et al. Soft-tissue masses: diagnosis using MR imaging. *AJR Am J Roentgenol* 1989;153(3):541-7.

2.5. Branchial Cleft Cyst

Branchial cleft cyst is also known as branchial cyst or lateral cervical cyst. There are four main theories about the origins of branchial cleft cysts; i.e., the branchial apparatus theory, cervical sinus theory, thymopharyngeal ductal theory, and inclusion theory [1]. In the inclusion theory, the cyst epithelium arises from the lymph node squamous epithelium; therefore, branchial cleft cysts are also known as lymphoepithelial cysts [1]. Branchial cleft cysts that develop in the second branchial arch often arise unilaterally from the neck in the anterior border of the sternocleidomastoid muscle [2]. Branchial cleft cysts also occur at other sites including the parotid gland, pharyngeal region, etc., although their occurrence at these sites is rare [2-9]. Branchial cleft cysts tend to occur in late childhood or early adulthood and display no sex predilection. Their characteristic clinical symptom is a soft and sessile swelling, which is usually painless. Histopathologically, the cyst walls of branchial cleft cysts are thin and lined with a stratified squamous epithelium overlying lymphoid tissue.

CT and MRI are useful modalities for diagnosing branchial cleft cysts as they develop in soft tissues. CT and MR images of branchial cleft cysts reflect the fact that their interiors mostly consist of fluid retaining areas; i.e., the central zone of the lesion shows homogeneous isodensity compared with that of the surrounding muscles on CT images (Figure 2.5.3) and homogenous hypointensity on T1WI and homogenous hyperintensity on T2WI (and STIR images). On CE-CT and CE-T1WI, the walls of branchial cleft cysts are usually thin and display rim enhancement or no enhancement after the administration of contrast medium (Figure 2.5.1, 2, 4)[10, 11].

The differential diagnoses of brachial cleft cysts include vascular malformations and neoplastic lesions (e.g., lipoma, schwannoma, and salivary gland tumors). MR imaging produces more helpful information for distinguishing branchial cleft cysts from other lesions, especially neoplastic lesions, than CT due to its superior soft tissue contrast. As another differential diagnosis for branchial cleft cyst, squamous cell carcinoma arising from the cyst wall should also be considered. The development of carcinoma from a branchial cleft cyst, which is known as bronchogenic carcinoma, is rare, and it appears as an eccentrically located nodule within the walls of the cyst on CT images [12-15].

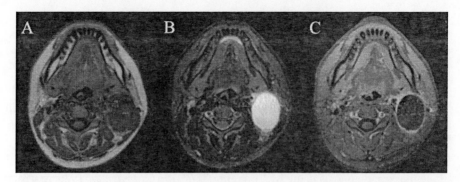

Figure 2.5.1. MR images of a branchial cleft cyst in the left lateral neck region of a 20-year-old female. Axial MR images of a branchial cleft cyst in the left lateral region showed a cystic mass that displayed almost homogeneous isointensity on T1WI (A) and heterogeneous marked hyperintensity on STIR images (B). The central zone of the cystic mass did not show any enhancement, whereas the peripheral zone showed marked enhancement on axial CE-T1WI (C).

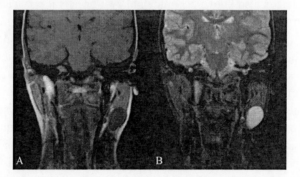

Figure 2.5.2. MR images of a branchial cleft cyst in the left lateral neck region of a 10-year-old female. Coronal T1WI (A) of a branchial cleft cyst in the left lateral region showed an oval mass that displayed almost homogeneous isointensity. STIR images displayed an oval mass that demonstrated almost heterogeneous hyperintensity (B).

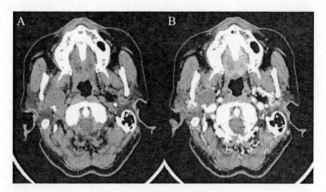

Figure 2.5.3. CT images of a branchial cleft cyst in the right masticator space of a 73-year-old female. An axial CT image showed an oval mass that displayed homogeneous hypodensity in the right masticator space (A). On a CE-CT image (B), the central zone of the lesion did not show any enhancement, whereas the peripheral zone did.

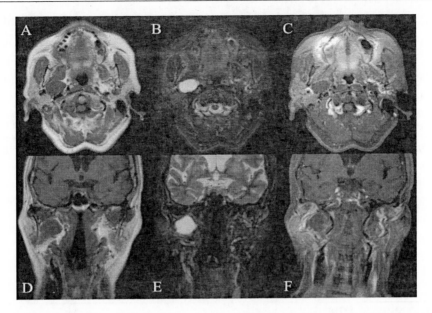

Figure 2.5.4. MR images of a branchial cleft cyst in the right masticator space of a 73-year-old female. Axial and coronal T1WI demonstrated an oval mass in the right masticator space that displayed homogeneous isointensity (A, D), and the peripheral zone of the lesion was enhanced on CE-T1WI (C, F). The central zone of the lesion showed homogeneous hyperintensity on axial and coronal T2WI (B, E).

References

[1]   King ES. The lateral lympho-epithelial cyst of the neck; branchial cyst. *Aust N Z J Surg* 1949 ;19(2):109-21, illust.

[2]   Agaton-Bonilla FC, Gay-Escoda C. Diagnosis and treatment of branchial cleft cysts and fistulae. A retrospective study of 183 patients. *Int J Oral Maxillofac Surg* 1996 ;25(6):449-52.

[3]   Bernier JL, Bhaskar SN. Lymphoepithelial lesions of salivary glands; histogenesis and classification based on 186 cases. *Cancer* 1958; 11(6):1156-79.

[4]   Bhaskar SN, Bernier JL. Histogenesis of branchial cysts; a report of 468 cases. *Am J Pathol* 1959;35(2):407-43.

[5]   Little JW, Rickles NH. The histogenesis of the branchial cyst. *Am J Pathol* 1967 ;50(3):533-47.

[6]   Shaheen OH. Two cases of bilateral branchiogenic cysts of the nasopharynx. *J Laryngol Otol* 1961;75:182-6.

[7]   Taylor JN, Burwell RG. Branchiogenic nasopharyngeal cysts. *J Laryngol Otol* 1954 ;68(10):667-79.

[8]   Piccin O, Cavicchi O, Caliceti U. Branchial cyst of the parapharyngeal space: report of a case and surgical approach considerations. *Oral Maxillofac Surg* 2008 Dec;12(4):215-7.

[9]   Shin JH, Lee HK, Kim SY, Park HW, Khang SK, Choi CG, et al. Parapharyngeal second branchial cyst manifesting as cranial nerve palsies: MR findings. *AJNR Am J Neuroradiol* 2001;22(3):510-2.

[10] Curtin HD. *Head and neck imaging.* 4th ed. St. Louis: Mosby: 2003.

[11] Koeller KK, Alamo L, Adair CF, Smirniotopoulos JG. Congenital cystic masses of the neck: radiologic-pathologic correlation. *Radiographics* 1999;19(1):121-46; quiz 52-3.

[12] Martin H, Morfit HM, Ehrlich H. The case for branchiogenic cancer (malignant branchioma). Ann Surg 1950;132(5):867-87.

[13] Khafif RA, Prichep R, Minkowitz S. Primary branchiogenic carcinoma. Head Neck 1989;11(2):153-63.

[14] Bhanote M, Yang GC. Malignant first branchial cleft cysts presented as submandibular abscesses in fine-needle aspiration: report of three cases and review of literature. Diagn Cytopathol 2008;36(12):876-81.

[15] Roche JP, Younes MN, Funkhouser WK, Weissler MC. Branchiogenic carcinoma of a first branchial cleft cyst. Otolaryngology--head and neck surgery : official journal of American Academy of Otolaryngology-*Head and Neck Surgery* 2010;143(1):167-8, 8 e1.

2.6. Thyroglossal Duct Cyst

Thyroglossal duct cysts, which are congenital cysts, are remnants of the embryonic thyroglossal duct. Thyroglossal duct cysts represent approximately 70% of all congenital cysts of the neck and present in the first three decades of life [1]. Thyroglossal duct cysts commonly occur along the midline (anywhere from the tongue to the thyroid gland). Furthermore, they can be located anterior or posterior to the hyoid bone or even within it because the thyroglossal duct is closely associated with the hyoid bone [2]. Regarding the localization of thyroglossal duct cysts, most (65%) occur in the infrahyoid neck, and the other sites include the suprahyoid neck (20%) and sites at the level of the hyoid bone (15%) [2, 3].

Thyroglossal duct cysts usually present as a painless palpable midline neck mass that is located at or below the level of the hyoid bone. Although thyroglossal duct cysts usually move upwards during swallowing or protrusion of the tongue, they are not usually associated with neck or throat pain, or dysphagia. Histopathologically, the cyst walls of thyroglossal duct cysts are lined by a diverse epithelium; i.e., a columnar, cuboidal, non-keratinized stratified squamous epithelium [4].

CT and MRI are useful modalities for diagnosing thyroglossal duct cysts due to the fact that they occur in soft tissues. On CT, thyroglossal duct cysts demonstrate a well-defined mass that displays homogenous hypodensity to that of the muscles and is located in an anterior midline or paramidline region of the neck. On CE-CT, the peripheral zone of the lesion (cyst wall) shows rim (capsular) enhancement. On MRI, thyroglossal duct cysts appear as a mass that displays homogeneous hypo- to isointensity on T1WI and hyperintensity on T2WI (STIR images) (Figure 2.6.1) [5]. CE-T1WI show thin peripheral enhancement of the mass similar to CE-CT images. The differential diagnoses of thyroglossal duct cyst include epidermoid/dermoid cyst, branchial cleft cyst, thyroid cyst, lymphatic malformations, and ranula [1-3, 6-12]. As another differential diagnosis, carcinoma arising from the cyst wall of a thyroglossal duct cyst should be considered, although the latter lesion is rare (accounting for less than 1% of cysts) [13]. Such carcinomas often display an enhanced mural nodule or calcification within the cyst wall on CT images [14].

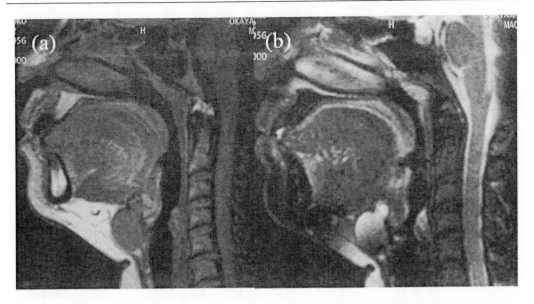

Figure 2.6.1. MR images of a thyroglossal duct cyst in a 43-year-old female. Sagittal MR images of a thyroglossal duct cyst of the anterior neck showing a cystic mass (arrows) that displays almost homogeneous isointensity on T1WI (A) and hyperintensity on T2WI (B). Adapted from reference no.5 (Asaumi J et al. Assessment of lesions arising or extending in the submental region with magnetic resonance imaging. Oral Radiol 2005;21:6–13).

References

[1]   al-Dousary S. Current management of thyroglossal-duct remnant. *J Otolaryngol* 1997;26(4):259-65.

[2]   Bourjat P, Cartier J, Woerther JP. Thyroglossal duct cyst in hyoid bone: CT confirmation. *J Comput Assist Tomogr* 1988;12(5):871-3.

[3]   Imhof H, Czerny C, Hormann M, Krestan C. Tumors and tumor-like lesions of the neck: from childhood to adult. *Eur Radiol* 2004;14 Suppl 4:L155-65.

[4]   Ward PH, Strahan RW, Acquarelli M, Harris PF. The many faces of cysts of the thyroglossal duct. Trans Am Acad Ophthalmol Otolaryngol 1970;74(2):310-8.

[5]   Asaumi J, Yanagi Y, Hisatomi M, Konouchi H, Matsuzaki H, Kishi K. Assessment of lesions arising or extending in the submental region with magnetic resonance imaging. *Oral Radiol* 2005;21:6–13. DOI 10.1007/s11282-004-0021-0

[6]   Koch BL. Cystic malformations of the neck in children. *Pediatr Radiol* 2005; 35(5):463-77.

[7]   Sari M, Baylancicek S, Inanli S, Sehitoglu MA. Unusual presentation and location of thyroglossal duct cyst in a child. Otolaryngology--head and neck surgery: official journal of American Academy of Otolaryngology-*Head and Neck Surgery* 2007;136(5):854-5.

[8]   Acierno SP, Waldhausen JH. Congenital cervical cysts, sinuses and fistulae. *Otolaryngol Clin North Am* 2007;40(1):161-76, vii-viii.

[9]   King AD, Ahuja AT, Mok CO, Metreweli C. MR imaging of thyroglossal duct cysts in adults. *Clin Radiol* 1999;54(5):304-8.

[10]   Lanzieri CF. Head and neck case of the day. Thyroglossal duct cyst. *AJR Am J Roentgenol* 1997;169(1):276, 9-80.

[11]   Vazquez E, Enriquez G, Castellote A, Lucaya J, Creixell S, Aso C, et al. US, CT, and MR imaging of neck lesions in children. *Radiographics* 1995;15(1):105-22.

[12]   Weber AL, Randolph G, Aksoy FG. The thyroid and parathyroid glands. CT and MR imaging and correlation with pathology and clinical findings. *Radiol Clin North Am* 2000;38(5):1105-29.

[13]   Reede DL, Bergeron RT, Som PM. CT of thyroglossal duct cysts. *Radiology* 1985;157(1):121-5.

[14]   Branstetter BF, Weissman JL, Kennedy TL, Whitaker M. The CT appearance of thyroglossal duct carcinoma. *AJNR Am J Neuroradiol* 2000;21(8):1547-50.

2.7. Ranula

A ranula is a mucous retention cyst or mucocele arising in the sublingual or submandibular space. The pathogenesis of ranula involves the extravasation of saliva from a damaged salivary duct or sublingual gland [1]. As the cyst wall consists of reactive fibrosis without an epithelial lining, ranulas are classified as pseudocysts. Ranulas can be divided into simple ranulas and plunging ranulas according to their growth pattern. The sublingual space and submandibular space are separated by the mylohyoid muscle. When a ranula is contained within the sublingual space, it is referred to as a simple ranula. Simple ranulas appear as a swelling on one side of the floor of the mouth [2] (Figure 2.7.1). Since epidermoid and dermoid cysts occur along the midline of the floor of the mouth, they can be distinguished from ranulas [3]. When a ranula extends below the mylohyoid muscle, it is classified as a plunging ranula, and surgical treatment is more difficult for such lesions than for simple ranulas. In recent years, various treatments have been reported, and surgical procedures for simple and plunging ranulas that do not involve excision of the sublingual gland have also been reported [4-6]. Therefore, it is important to assess the extent of a ranula during diagnostic imaging.

As ranulas are soft tissue lesions, CT, MRI, and ultrasonography are useful for their imaging diagnosis. CT and MR imaging are particularly useful for evaluating the spatial relationship between a ranula and the floor of the mouth. On CT, ranulas typically appear as well-defined homogeneous, low-density lesions (Figure 2.7.2). CT might also reveal defects in the mylohyoid muscle and deviation of the tongue and submandibular gland. However, some small simple ranulas can not be detected by CT. As MR imaging provides better soft-tissue resolution than CT, it is useful for detecting small lesions. Moreover, in order to evaluate the reduction of a lesion brought about by treatments in which the sublingual gland is not excised, it s necessary to perform frequent evaluations. In such cases, MR imaging should be used in order to avoid frequent radiation exposure. MR images of ranulas display the same signal intensity as general cysts. The cystic cavities show homogeneous hypointensity on T1WI, homogeneous marked hyperintensity on T2WI and STIR images, and no enhancement (Figure 2.7.3).

As simple ranulas extend from the anterior to posterior region of the sublingual space, they show a well-defined round or oval shape. On the other hand, dermoid cysts and epidermoid cysts often occur in the medial sublingual space. Therefore, it is necessary to distinguish ranulas from these cysts. On CT and MRI, dermoid cysts typically look like inhomogeneous masses, which reflects the mixture of keratin and fat that they contain. These findings can be used to differentiate ranulas from other cysts, especially dermoid cysts. Since plunging ranulas extend into the submandibular space and other spaces beyond the mylohyoid muscle, it is difficult to obtain complete information about their three-dimensional structure (Figure 2.7.4). In CT or MR imaging, the identifying characteristic of a plunging ranula is the "tail sign"; i.e., the slight extension of a cyst in the submandibular space into the sublingual space [3] (Figure 2.'9.5). The "tail sign" displayed by plunging ranulas is easier to detect with MRI than CT.

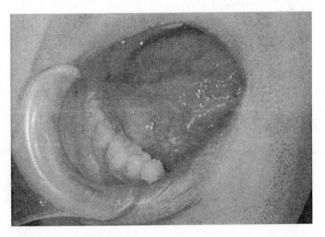

Figure 2.7.1. Photograph showing a swelling on the right side of the floor of the mouth of a 30-year-old male.

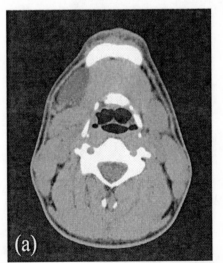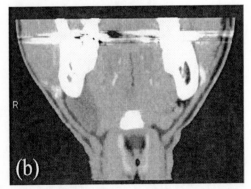

Figure 2.7.2. CT images showing a well-defined, homogeneous, low-density mass in a 31-year-old male. A coronal CT image reveals a cystic lesion located in the right submandibular space below the mylohyoid muscle.

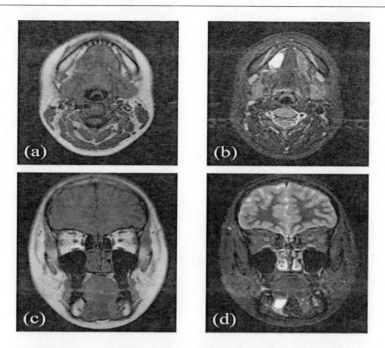

Figure 2.7.3. A simple ranula in a 17-year-old female. MR images reveal a small, well-defined, and oval shaped mass in the right sublingual space (a-d). The cystic lesion shows homogeneous hypointensity on axial and coronal T1WI (a, c) and homogeneous marked hyperintensity on axial and coronal STIR images (b, d).

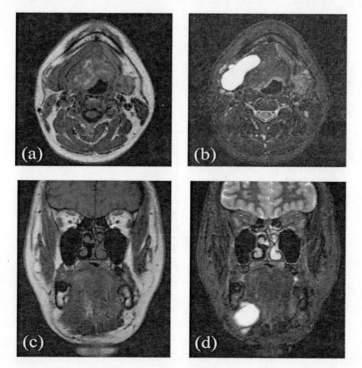

Figure 2.7.4. A plunging ranula in a 34-year-old male. MR images reveal a large, well-defined, and oval shaped mass in the right submandibular space (a-d). Coronal T1WI (c) and STIR images (d) are especially useful for depicting the spatial relationship between the lesion and the mylohyoid muscle.

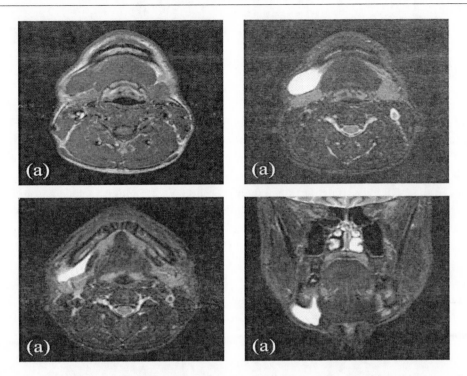

Figure 2.7.5. A plunging ranula in a 31-year-old male. Axial T1WI (a) and STIR images (b) reveal a cystic mass in the right submandibular space. The right submandibular gland has been deformed and pushed backwards by the progression of the lesion. Axial (c) and coronal (d) STIR images reveal that the lesion in the submandibular space extends into the sublingual space.

References

[1]   Bhaskar SN, Bolden TE, Weinmann JP. Pathogenesis of mucoceles. Journal of dental research. 1956;35:863-74.

[2]   La'porte SJ, Juttla JK, Lingam RK. Imaging the floor of the mouth and the sublingual space. Radiographics : a review publication of the Radiological Society of North America, Inc. 2011;31:1215-30.

[3]   Tohru KURABAYASHI, Shin Nakamura, Ichiro OGURA, Sasaki T. The sublingual and submandibular spaces. *Oral Radiology.* 2003;19:28-34.

[4]   Harrison JD. Modern management and pathophysiology of ranula: literature review. *Head & neck.* 2010;32:1310-20.

[5]   Baurmash HD. Marsupialization for treatment of oral ranula: a second look at the procedure. *Journal of oral and maxillofacial surgery : official journal of the American Association of Oral and Maxillofacial Surgeons.* 1992;50:1274-9.

[6]   Takagi S, Mizukawa N, Kimura T, Asaumi JI. Treatment of a plunging ranula with fenestration and continuous pressure. *The British journal of oral & maxillofacial surgery.* 2003;41:410-3.

3. OTHERS

3.1. Keratocystic Odontogenic Tumor

Keratocystic odontogenic tumors (KCOT) are benign unicystic or multicystic tumors of odontogenic origin that occur in the jawbone. The original designation of KCOT was odontogenic keratocyst (OKC), which indicated that they display benign behavior. However, in 2005 the WHO Working Group recommended the term KCOT as it better reflects the neoplastic nature of this lesion [1]. Although KCOT were newly classified as neoplastic lesions in the WHO classification, since their morphological findings include a cystic lesion, their differential radiographic diagnoses include other cystic lesions that affect the jawbone. In addition, because KCOT have a high recurrence rate, the strategy employed for their surgical management differs from those used for other cysts. Therefore, we also explain the imaging features of KCOT in this chapter.

Histopathologically, KCOT display a cystic form, which is lined by a characteristic parakeratinized stratified squamous epithelium. Exfoliated keratinous debris is stored in their cystic cavities [2]. In some KCOT, the connective tissue contains islands of epithelial tissue or separate daughter cysts.

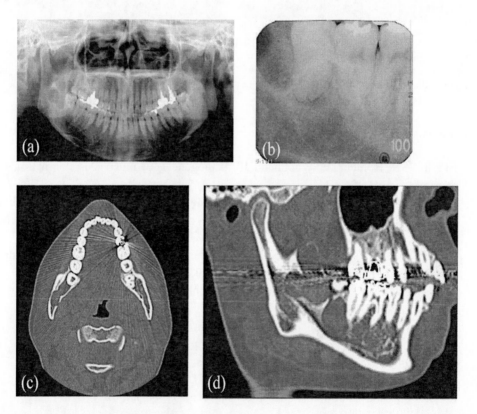

Figure 3.1.1. A 24-year-old female. Panoramic (a) and periapical radiographs (b) showed a well-defined multilocular radiolucent lesion with a smooth and sclerotic border on the right side of the mandible. Axial (c) and reconstructed sagittal CT images (d) revealed slight cortical expansion and the spatial relationship between the lesion and adjacent structures such as the mandibular canal and teeth.

Radiographically, KCOT show unilocular or multilocular areas of radiolucency with smooth and sclerotic borders. Furthermore, multilocular KCOT have undulating borders and arc-like internal septa (Figure 3.1.1-a, b). The adjacent teeth might be displaced, but root resorption rarely occurs. Although KCOT often involve an impacted tooth, there is no fixed pattern for the spatial relationship between the lesion and the impacted tooth. Unilocular KCOT need to be distinguished from radicular cysts, dentigerous cysts, and simple bone cysts (Figure 3.1.2a). When KCOT involve an impacted tooth, care must be taken to distinguish them from dentigerous cysts, which are characterized as including a tooth crown. The characteristic radiographic findings of multilocular KCOT are similar to those of ameloblastoma and simple bone cysts involving the alveolar septum. Thus, in conventional radiography, it is sometimes difficult to distinguish KCOT from other jawbone lesions.

CT scans might be helpful for detecting cortical expansion and the spatial relationship between the lesion and the impacted tooth (Figure 3.1.1c, d). The CT value of the cystic contents might also be useful in some cases. The CT values of general cystic fluid and solid tumor are about 0 to 30 HU and 40 to 80 HU, respectively. Since exfoliated keratinous debris is included in cystic contents of KCOT, its CT value ranges from about 20 to 45 HU.

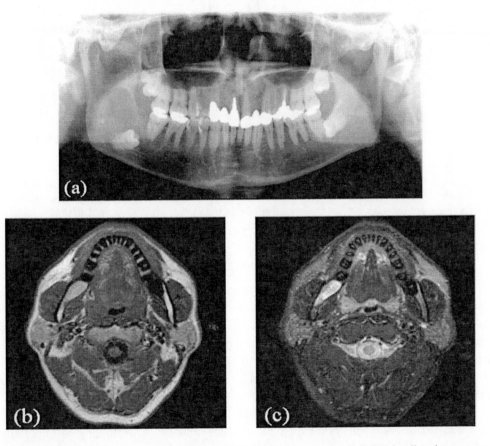

Figure 3.1.2. A 49-year-old male. A panoramic radiograph (a) shows a well-defined unilocular radiolucent lesion with an impacted tooth on the right side of the mandible. The cystic cavity displays hyperintensity on T1WI (b) and a heterogeneous mix of isointensity and marked hyperintensity on T2W.

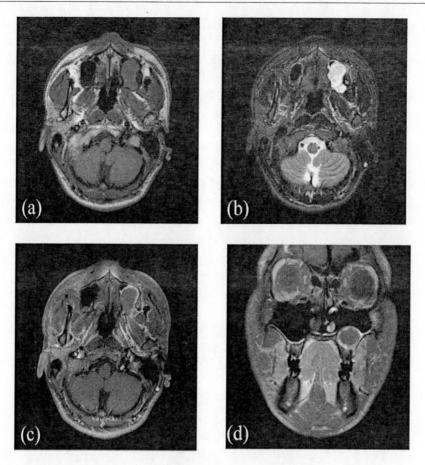

Figure 3.1.3. An 18-year-old male. Axial MR images demonstrated a unilocular lesion in the maxilla, which showed isointensity on T1WI (a) and a heterogeneous mix of iso- and marked hyperintensity on STIR images (b). The cystic cavity showed no enhancement on contrast-enhanced (CE)-T1WI (c, d). Axial (c) and coronal CE- T1WI (d) demonstrated that the cystic border displayed an uneven thickness of 1 mm or more.

MR imaging is also very useful for differentiating cystic lesions from solid tumors and evaluating their cystic contents. MR images of KCOT show characteristic findings (Figure 3.1.2b, c, 3-1)-3). Some or all of their cystic cavities show hyper- to isointensity on T1WI, heterogeneous iso- to marked hyperintensity on T2WI, and no enhancement. Their cyst borders show thin or thick rim enhancement. The cystic fluid of general cysts displays hypointensity on T1WI and marked hyperintensity on T2WI. Fat tissue, high-density protein solution, and areas of hemorrhaging display hyperintensity on T1WI. Thus, the hyperintensity observed in the cystic cavities of KCOT on T1WI reflects the fact that they contain a large amount of keratin [3-6].

In our previous study, which investigated 10 cases of unilocular KCOT, 70% showed higher signal intensity on T1WI than the masseter muscle. This finding is important for differentiating KCOT from other cysts. However, dentigerous cysts also show higher signal intensity on T1WI than the masseter muscle. Therefore, it might be difficult to differentiate KCOT from dentigerous cysts using T1WI. On the other hand, in an investigation of the thickness of the cystic border using CE-MR imaging, although KCOT and other cystic lesions displayed borders that were less than 3 mm thick, the borders of tumors that displayed cystic changes were not less than 3 mm thick. Furthermore, although the borders of other cystic lesions are uniform and less than 1 mm thick, the borders of some KCOT(s) are uneven and so are thicker than 1 mm in some areas (Figure 3d). When KCOT show these findings, they can be distinguished from dentigerous cysts.

In clinical imaging diagnosis, radiography is always performed before MRI. Dentigerous cysts are characterized by the presence of the crown of an unerupted tooth, and they can be diagnosed comparatively easily using radiography. Therefore, if MR imaging diagnosis based on the abovementioned findings and radiographic diagnosis are combined, highly accurate diagnostic imaging is possible.

CONCLUSION

This chapter showed that CT and MRI are able to offer information that aids the differential diagnosis of cysts and pseudocysts in the oral and maxillofacial region. Moreover, CT and MRI might also be useful for demonstrating the extent of lesions prior to surgery. CT and MRI are relatively non-invasive methods and although they are expensive and carry a risk of problems associated with radiation exposure they are sometimes necessary for differential diagnosis in the oral and maxillofacial region.

REFERENCES

[1]   Leon Barnes JWE, Peter Reichart, David Sidransky. WHO Classification of Tumours. *Pathology and Genetics of Head and Neck Tumours.* Lyon: IARC; 2005.

[2]   Shafer WG HM, Levy BM. *A textbook of oral pathology,* 3rd ed. . Philadelphia: Saunders WB; 1974.

[3]   Minami M, Kaneda T, Ozawa K, Yamamoto H, Itai Y, Ozawa M, et al. Cystic lesions of the maxillomandibular region: MR imaging distinction of odontogenic keratocysts and ameloblastomas from other cysts. *AJR American journal of roentgenology.* 1996;166:943-9.

[4]   Hisatomi M, Asaumi J, Konouchi H, Shigehara H, Yanagi Y, Kishi K. MR imaging of epithelial cysts of the oral and maxillofacial region. *European journal of radiology.* 2003;48:178-82.

[5]   Konouchi H, Asaumi J, Yanagi Y, Hisatomi M, Kawai N, Matsuzaki H, et al. Usefulness of contrast enhanced-MRI in the diagnosis of unicystic ameloblastoma. *Oral oncology.* 2006;42:481-6.

[6]   Janse van Rensburg L, Nortje CJ, Thompson I. Correlating imaging and histopathology of an odontogenic keratocyst in the nevoid basal cell carcinoma syndrome. *Dento maxillo facial radiology.* 1997;26:195-9.

In: Cysts: Causes, Diagnosis and Treatment Options
Editors: A. Mendes Ortiz and A. Jimenez Moreno

ISBN: 978-1-62081-315-7
© 2012 Nova Science Publishers, Inc.

Chapter 2

INFLAMMATORY ODONTOGENIC CYSTS

Louis M. Lin, Paul A. Rosenberg and Domenico Ricucci

Department of Endodontics, New York University College of Dentistry, New York,
New York, US

ABSTRACT

A radicular cyst is a pathologic cavity partially or completely lined by epithelium in an area of apical periodontitis. It is caused by infection of the root canal system, which results in an immuno-inflammatory response of the periapical tissues. A radicular cyst is presumably formed by inflammatory proliferation of epithelial cell rests in an area of apical periodontitis. Radicular cysts can be categorized into pocket and true cysts. Clinically, it is not possible to make a definitive diagnosis of a radicular cyst. The final conclusive diagnosis of a radicular cyst can only be made through histological examination of biopsy specimens. Radicular cysts [pocket and true] are of inflammatory origin and are not developmental or neoplastic. As in other infectious diseases, they should be able to regress after elimination of infection, possibly by the mechanism of apoptosis or programmed cell death. Since radicular cysts cannot be diagnosed clinically, all cyst-like inflammatory periapical lesions should be treated initially by conservative procedures, such as non-surgical root canal therapy or a decompression technique. If large cyst-like periapical lesions are treated surgically, recurrence will not occur even if the epithelial lining is not completely enucleated. Failure of radicular cysts to regress after non-surgical or surgical treatment is due to persistent intraradicular infection or reinfection of involved teeth and not due to a self-sustaining nature of the cysts.

INTRODUCTION

A cyst is a pathologic cavity partially or completely lined by epithelium, which can occur in the soft or hard tissues of the body. According to the World Health Organization, cysts in the oral cavity are classified as developmental, neoplastic, and inflammatory origin [Main1985, Kramer and Pindborg 1992]. The cause of neoplastic cysts [e.g., odontogenic keratocyst] is not clear although mutation of specific genes has been suggested [Barreto et al.

2000, Collins et al. 2004, Barnes et al. 2005, Li 2011]. Developmental cysts [e.g., dentigerous cyst] are due to anomalous tissue formations [Kramer and Pindborg 1992, Neville et al. 2009]. In contrast, the etiology of inflammatory cysts [radicular cyst, residual cyst] is well established [Nair 2004]. In this chapter, discussion of cysts will be focused on inflammatory odontogenic cysts, namely radicular and residual cysts.

A radicular cyst is a pathologic cavity partially or completely lined by epithelium in an area of apical periodontitis. It is a product of apical periodontitis. A residual cyst is considered to be a radicular cyst that remains in the jawbone after removal of the involved tooth [Neville et al. 2009]. In fact, it is not known if a cyst-like periapical lesion associated with an endodontically involved tooth is actually a radicular cyst because after tooth extraction a biopsy is not usually performed to confirm the disease entity. A radicular cyst is presumably formed by inflammatory hyperplasia or proliferation of the epithelial cell rests of Malassez in an area of apical periodontitis, which is caused by root canal infection [Nair 2004, Lin et al. 2007]. Epithelial cell rests in the periodontal ligament appear to maintain the characteristic properties of stem cells, i.e. self-renewal and differentiation [Lin et al. 2007]. In the steady state, epithelial cell rests remain quiescent but can be stimulated to proliferate by pro-inflammatory mediators, pro-inflammatory cytokines and growth factors released by the host's immuno-inflammatory cells in apical periodontitis lesions [Lin et al. 2007].

Several theories concerning radicular cyst formation have been proposed [Shear 1963, Oehlers 1970, Ten Cate 1972, Valderhaug 1974, Summers 1974, Torabinejad 1983, Lin et al. 2007, Nair et al. 2008]. Nevertheless, the exact mechanism of development of radicular cyst in humans is still not fully understood. Definitive diagnosis of radicular cysts can only be made through histological examination of biopsy specimens [Nair 1998, Ricucci et al. 2006b].

Similar to all infectious diseases, radicular cysts and residual cysts are of immuno-inflammatory origin, therefore they should be able to resolve or heal, possibly by the mechanism of apoptosis or programmed cell death after elimination of infection by non-surgical root canal therapy [Lin et al. 2009]. A decompression technique may be used as an alternate treatment of choice rather than surgery when treating large inflammatory periapical cystic lesions in the maxilla or mandible in order to avoid injury to the adjacent vital teeth or anatomical vital structures [Neaverth and Burg 1982, Rees 1997, Oztan 2002, Tandri 2010].

If radicular cysts are treated surgically, recurrence will not occur even if the epithelial lining is not completely enucleated [Lin et al. 1996]. It is important to note that radicular cysts are not neoplastic lesions, which must be completely removed surgically to prevent recurrence. Failure of non-surgical or surgical endodontic treatment of radicular cysts is due to persistent intraradicular infection or reinfection or possibly extraradicular infection of the involved tooth [Siquera 2001, Ricucci et al. 2005, Ricucci et al. 2009, Ricucci and Siqueira 2010] and not due to the self-sustaining nature of radicular cysts [Lin et al. 2009].

EPIDEMIOLOGY

Radicular cysts are associated with infected necrotic teeth with apical periodontitis [Nair 2004]. They occur more frequently in the maxilla than in mandible [Bhaskar 1968, Nakamura et al. 1995, Koseoglu et al. 2004] and are more common in men than in women [Shear 1963,

Bhaskar 1966, Koseoglu et al. 2004. The most frequent occurrence of radicular cysts is in patients in their third decade of life [Shear 1963, Bhaskar 1966, Nakamura et al. 1995]. The prevalence of radicular cysts reported in the literature varies considerably from 6 to 55% inareas of apical periodontitis [Seltzer et al. 1967, Bhaskar 1966, Mortensen et al. 1970, Block et al. 1976, Simon 1980, Stockdale and Chandler 1988, Spatafore et al. 1990, Lin et al. 1991, Nobuhara and Del Rio 1993, Nair 1996, Sanchis et al. 1998, Ricucci et al. 2005, Love and Firth 2009, Schulz et al. 2009]. This wide range of discrepancy is probably due to incompletely removed biopsy specimens and the absence of standardized criteria of histopathological interpretation of cysts [Nair 1998]. The prevalence of radicular cysts probably ranges between 15 to 20%.

ETIOLOGY

A radicular cyst is formed in an area of apical periodontitis, which is caused by pulpal infection [Kakehashi et al. 1965, Möller et al. 1981]. When pulp tissue is infected, a complex immuno-inflammatory response occurs in the pulp tissue [Hahn and Liewehr 2007a, 2007b]. The response exemplifies the battle between the host's programmed defenses and tissue destruction induced by bacterial infection. Unfortunately, the potential of infected pulp tissue to recover is minimal because the pulp tissue is enclosed in rigid dentin walls, which hinders dissipation of increased pulpal interstitial pressure during pulpal inflammation [Heyeraas and Berggreen 1999]. In addition, the access of cellular and humoral components of innate and adaptive immune defense mechanisms carried by the circulation to the pulp tissue is restricted by small apical foramina. Eventually, pulpal infection/inflammation gradually spreads apically into the periapical tissues and causes apical periodontitis (Kovacevic et al. 2008).

The mechanism of the immuno-inflammatory response that takes place in the periapical tissues is similar to that in the pulpal tissue. In pulpitis, the loose fibrous connective tissue is affected, while in apical periodontitis, both fibrous [periodontal ligament] and hard [alveolar bone] connective tissues are involved. Apical periodontitis can be classified as an apical granuloma, apical abscess, and apical cyst or radicular cyst [Nair et al. 1996, Ricucci et al. 2006, Neville et al. 2009].

PATHOGENESIS

The most conspicuous histological features of apical periodontitis are destruction of apical alveolar bone and replacement of periapical tissues by inflamed tissue [Figure 1]. Apical bone destruction is caused by a complex network of interaction involving osteoblasts, osteoclast progenitor cells, growth factors, cytokines and innate and adaptive immune cells [Stashenko and Yu 1989, Stashenko 1990, Wang and Stashenko 1991, Wallström et al. 1993, Tani-Ishii et al. 1995, Fouad 1997, Kawashima and Stashenko 1999, Teitelbaum 2000, Colic et al. 2009]. Approximately 52% of inflammatory periapical lesions from extracted teeth showed proliferation of epithelial cell rests of Malassez [ERM] [Nair et al. 1996].

ERM are the remnants of disintegrated Hertwig's epithelial root sheath during tooth development and are present in the periodontal ligament around all mature teeth [Reeve et al.

1962, Valderhaug and Zander 1967, Seltzer 1988, Nanci 2007] [Figure 2]. Epithelial proliferation in an area of apical periodontitis is a form of pathologic hyperplasia. Inflammation-induced epithelial proliferation is also seen in many infected/inflamed epithelial tissues, such as bronchial epithelium [Ricciardolo et al. 2003], gastrointestinal tract epithelium [MacDonald 1992, Berstad et al. 1997], genitourinary tract epithelium [Shankar et al. 2001] and lung [Haegens et al. 2005].

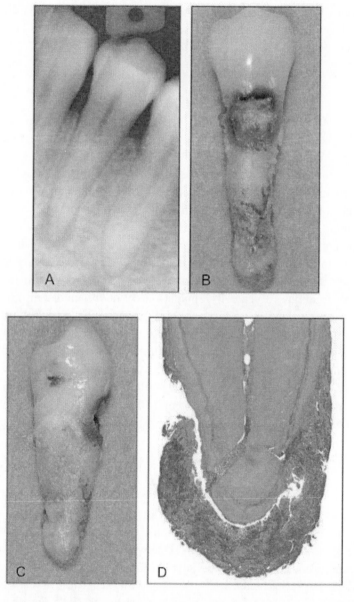

Figure 1. A. Radiograph of mandibular left first premolar showing cervical caries and an apical osteolytic lesion. B-C. Buccal and mesial views of the extracted tooth with the pathologic periapical tissue remained attached to the apex at extraction. D. Section showing the root canal with two apical ramifications and attached periapical tissue; one apical ramification on the right and the other on the left side of the apex. Note that the tissue in the most apical part of the left apical ramification is vital. The periapical bone is replaced by inflamed tissue. The empty space between the inflamed periapical tissue

and the apex is an artifact. There is no epithelium in this lesion, and the histological diagnosis is periapical granuloma (H and E, original magnification ×16).

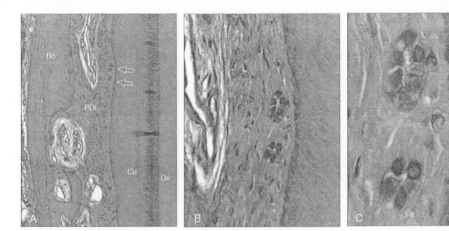

Figure 2. A. Histology of normal periodontal ligament. From right to left are dentin, cementum, periodontal ligament, and alveolar bone. Arrows indicate two small groups of cells in the PDL, close to cementum (H and E, original magnification ×100). B-C. High magnifications showing that these structures are nests of epithelial cell rests of Malassez surrounded by basement membrane (H and E, original magnification ×400 and ×1000). De, dentin; Ce, cementum; PDL, periodontal ligament; Bo, alveolar bone.

Epithelial cells proliferate in an area of apical periodontitis as a three-dimensional structure. They form irregular strands or islands of epithelium similar to arcades, which surround cores of vascular connective tissue infiltrated with varying degrees of inflammatory cells [Seltzer et al. 1969, Nair et al. 1996, Ricucci et al. 2006] [Figure 3]. The irregular strands of epithelium are often connected and may appear as a cyst in a two-dimensional histological structure. In an infected/inflamed respiratory tract or gastrointestinal tract, the epithelial cells proliferate and increase thickness of the epithelium. It has been postulated that epithelial proliferation in these tissues physically prevents penetration of irritants, such as bacteria into the underlying connective tissue, although the biological function of epithelium, for example, loss of cilia or microvilli, may be compromised [Kumar et al. 2009].

Nevertheless, it is not known biologically why epithelial cell rests proliferate irregularly in an area of apical periodontitis. They do not seem to serve any protective mechanism for the periapical tissues. Nair et al. [1996] showed that bacteria in the apical root canal might be blocked by epithelial plug-like growth into the apical foramen in apical periodontitis with epithelial proliferation.

Similar to the basal stem cells in the skin or stem cells in the bulge of hair follicles, epithelial cell rests in the periodontal ligament are uni-potent stem cells [Lin et al. 2007]. They appear to maintain characteristic properties of stem cells, i.e. self-renewal and differentiation. Epithelial cell rests can only differentiate into an epithelial cell lineage. In a normal micro-environmental niche, epithelial cell rests are in a steady-state condition that is mitotically quiescent [McHugh and Zander 1965, Valderhaug and Nylen 1966]. However, they can be stimulated to enter the cell cycle and start to proliferate upon receiving appropriate inductive signals, such as growth factors, cytokines, extracellular matrix, and cell surface adhesion molecules in the area of apical periodontitis [Lin et al. 2007].

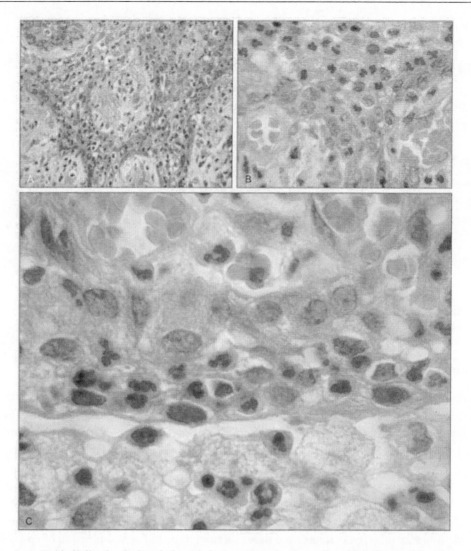

Figure 3. A. Epithelialized apical periodontitis lesion. Strands of arcading epithelium surround cores of connective tissue infiltrated with inflammatory cells (Masson Trichrome, original magnification ×400). B-C. High magnification of epithelial strands infiltrated by many polymorphonuclear leukocytes (Masson Trichrome, original magnification ×1000).

During periapical inflammation, intracanal bacteria release toxins and metabolic by-products into the periapical tissues. In addition, many of the host's cells such as polymorphonuclear leukocytes, macrophages,,lymphocytes, natural killer cells, fibroblasts, dendritic cells and osteoclasts participating in immuno-inflammatory responses in the periapical tissues release inflammatory mediators, pro-inflammatory cytokines and growth factors. Endotoxin and cytokines have been reported to play a role in the development of odontogenic cysts [Meghji et al. 1996]. Elevation of the intracellular level of cyclic adenosine monophophate caused by prostaglandins [PGE$_2$] appeared to stimulate the growth of epithelial cell rests [Brunett 1984]. Interleukin [IL]-1, IL-6 and keratinocyte growth factor [KGF] have been shown to stimulate epithelial cell proliferation [Sauder 1989, Grossman et al. 1989, Chedid et al. 1994, Meghji et al. 1996]. Epidermal growth factor [EGF] receptors are expressed by epithelial cells in the normal periodontal ligament and in odontogenic cysts [Thesleff 1987, Nordlund et al. 1991,

Irwin et al. 1991, Li et al. 1993] and are upregulated in periapical inflammation [Irwin et al. 1991, Lin et al. 1996]. Transforming growth factor alpha [TGF-α] is also a potent epithelial cell mitogen and shares the same receptor and biological activities with EGF [Keutteke and Lee 1990]. It was suggested that PGE_2, IL-1, IL-6, tumor necrosis factor [TNF], and TGF-a might modulate the biological activities of the EGF receptors or upregulate EGF receptor gene expression by influencing transcription factors, thus enhancing ligand-receptor binding affinity and stimulating proliferation of epithelial cell rests [Irwin et al. 1991, Lin et al. 1996, Chang et al. 1996]. Gao et al. [1996] showed that pro-inflammatory cytokines could indirectly stimulate proliferation and growth of the epithelial cell rests by inducing KGF expression in the stromal fibroblasts. It has been shown that Th2 and Foxp3$^+$ T regulatory cells and their cytokines might be involved in the development of radicular cysts [Ihan and Ihan 2009, Marcal et al. 2010, Teixeira-Salum et al. 2010]. Proliferation of epithelial cell rests in an area of apical periodontitis has the potential to develop into a radicular cyst.

Several theories have been proposed as the possible cause of radicular cyst formation. The nutritional deficiency theory assumes that if epithelial islands kept growing into a three-dimensional ball mass, the central cells of the epithelial mass would move further away from their source of nutrition and undergo necrosis and liquefaction degeneration. The necrotic products would attract neutrophilic leukocytes into the necrotic area and form micro-abscesses. The micro-cavities would coalesce to form a cystic cavity lined by stratified squamous epithelium [Ten Cate1972]. However, in psoriasis and pyostomatitis vegetans, microabscesses are formed within the epithelium [Kumar et al. 2009, Femiano et al. 2009] but cysts would not form in these two lesions. In addition, epithelial islands or strands are frequently infiltrated with polymorphonuclear leukocytes [Seltzer 1988, Nair et al. 1996, Ricucci et al. 2006b, Lin et al. 2007] [Figure 3] and cell necrosis is not often seen in the center of epithelial islands or strands.

The abscess theory postulated that if an abscess cavity was formed in connective tissue, epithelial cells would proliferate and line the abscess cavity because of their inherent tendency to cover exposed connective tissue surface [Oehlers 1970, Summers 1974]. In histological sections of apical periodontitis lesions, it is possible to observe microabscesses in fibrovascular connective tissue at varying distances from proliferating epithelium and sometimes in the fibrovascular tissue surrounded by proliferating epithelial strands (Figure 4). Nevertheless, in dermatitis herpetiformis, micro-abscesses are often formed in subepithelial connective tissue [Kumar et al. 2009] but the overlying skin epithelial cells would not proliferate and line the abscess cavity. Experimentally, inflammatory cysts have been produced in 2 of 16 animals by implanting tissue cages consisting of sterile perforated cylinders of Teflon in the back of rats. The cages were inoculated with cultured epithelial cells obtained from non-autogenous palatal gingival biopsies and *Fusobacterium nucleatum* [Nair et al. 2008]. However, it is not known if the events associated with inflammatory cyst formation induced in rats are similar to that of radicular cyst formation in an area of apical periodontitis in humans.

Living tissue cannot tolerate an abscess caused by infection [Majno and Joris 2004, Kumar et al. 2009]. In the human body, the normal or commensal microbial flora colonize in tissues in contact or in communication with the external environment, namely the skin, eye, mouth, upper respiratory tract, gastrointestinal tract, and genitourinary tracts [Strohl et al. 2001, Mims et al. 2004]. Normally, the internal organs and systems are sterile [Strohl et al. 2001, Mims et al. 2004].

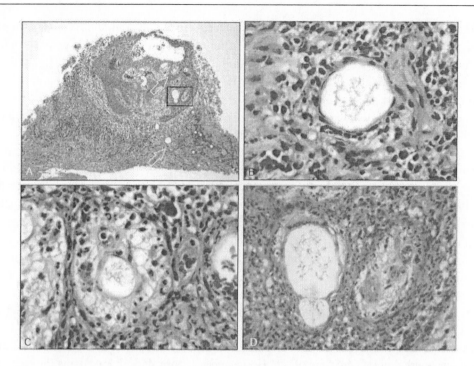

Figure 4. A. Epithelial proliferation in an apical periodontitis lesion (H and E, original magnification ×50). B. Magnification of the cavity indicated by the lower open arrow in A. A microcavity contains debris in connective tissue surrounded by a dense concentration of chronic inflammatory cells (H and E, original magnification ×400). C. Magnification of the area indicated by the upper open arrow in A. A microcavity contains debris in the connective tissue core surrounded by epithelium (H and E, original magnification ×400). D. Area demarcated by the rectangle in A. Two microcavities contain debris in the proliferating epithelium infiltrated by inflammatory cells (H and E, original magnification ×400). Considerations. Microcavities are observed in the same apical periodontitis lesion; in the inflamed connective tissue far from the lesion, in the connective tissue core surrounded by epithelium, and in the epithelial strands, demonstrating that the cavitation necessary for cyst formation may take place both in epithelium and connective tissue. Reprinted with permission from: Ricucci D. Patologia e Clinica Endodontica. Edizioni Martina, Bologna, Italy, 2009.

The bacteria reside only on the surface of epithelium and not in the subepithelial connective tissue. There is no biological evidence that epithelial cells are capable of eliminating bacteria, or an abscess. When an abscess occurs in living tissues, it is surrounded by granulation tissue, which is protective and equipped with powerful innate and adaptive immune defense mechanisms consisting of cellular and humoral components to wall off and to eliminate abscess [Majno and Joris 2004, Kumar et al. 2009]. These two defense mechanisms are highly effective in repair and/or regeneration of the tissue during wound healing. It is possible that when an abscess is formed in an area of apical periodontitis, the abscess is initially surrounded by granulation tissue and subsequently epithelial cells in the granulation tissue proliferate and completely enclose the abscess as a ball-like mass. Biologically, it is unlikely that the epithelial cell rests could proliferate and directly surround an abscess without prior granulation tissue formation unless the patients have compromised defense mechanisms. In fact, epithelial proliferation is rarely seen in an area of apical periodontitis with abscess formation but is seen more often in an area of chronic apical granulomas. Furthermore, the patients who develop radicular cysts in an area of apical periodontitis have not been shown to be deficient in innate and/or adaptive immune defense mechanisms.

The theory of merging of epithelial strands hypothesizes that if epithelial strands or islands proliferated, merged and formed a three-dimensional ball-like mass, the connective tissue trapped inside the ball-like mass would degenerate and a cyst would be formed (Lin et al. 2007). There is no direct evidence from histological observations of radicular cysts to support this hypothesis. As described previously, proliferating epithelial strands may completely surround a core of vital connective tissue and can look like a cyst in two-dimensional histological sections. Nevertheless, the core of connective tissue does not often show signs of degeneration.

The exact mechanism of radicular cyst formation in an area of apical periodontitis in humans is still not fully understood. Similar to proliferation of irregular epithelial strands or islands in an area of apical periodontitis, it is also not known why a radicular cyst, especially a true cyst, is formed in an area of apical periodontitis. It has been postulated that an epithelium-lined pouch-like extension of the root canal space of pocket cysts has much in common with a marginal periodontal pocket in acting as a death trap and garbage bag for the externalized and dying neutrophils (Nair et al. 1996). However, a marginal periodontal pocket is due to apical migration of junctional epithelium caused by marginal periodontitis. Junctional epithelium is a normal component of periodontium and acts physically to prevent bacteria from the gingival sulcus or pocket from invading the subepithelial connective tissue. The epithelial lining of pocket cysts is due to proliferation of epithelial cell rests caused by apical periodontitis. Although epithelial cell rests are a normal component of periodontal ligament, they do not appear to provide physical protection for the periapical tissues.

PATHOLOGY

A radicular cyst is a pathologic cavity partially or completely lined by non-keratinized stratified squamous epithelium in an area of apical periodontitis [Figs. 5, 6]. Radicular cysts can be categorized into two types: pocket or bay cyst and true cyst (Simon 1980, Nair et al. 1996). A pocket cyst is defined as an epithelium-lined pathological cavity, which is open to the canal of the affected tooth (Simon 1980, Nair 1998) [Figure 6]. A true cyst is a chronic inflammatory lesion at the periapex that contains an epithelium lined, closed pathological cavity (Simon 1980, Nair 1988) [Figure 5]. The lumen of a true cyst does not open to the canal of an involved tooth. It must be emphasized that in histological sections, the difference between true and pocket cysts can only be made in teeth with a single root canal and ending with one apical foramen approximately at the root tip. However, in teeth where a single root canal ends with several minor ramifications at the apex, it is practically impossible to differentiate between true and pocket cysts [Figure 7]. At times, more than one radicular cyst may be formed in the same area of an apical periodontitis lesion (Ricucci et al. 2006] [Figure 8].

In active infection/inflammation, the epithelial lining of radicular cysts is thick and irregular and infiltrated by many inflammatory cells [Figure 9]. The epithelial cells of the

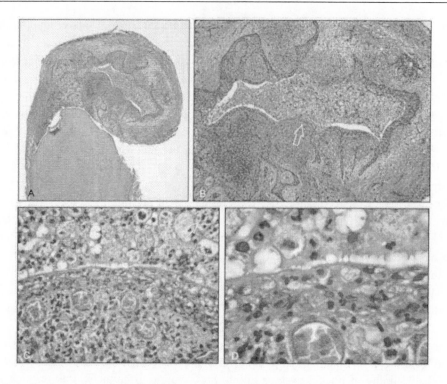

Figure 5. A. Cystic apical periodontitis lesion. Approximately at the center of the lesion, a pathologic cavity is completely lined by non-keratinized stratified squamous epithelium with irregular thickness and proliferation. It must be noted although the cyst lumen does not show communication with the root canal space in this section; the definitive diagnosis of a true cyst can be made only after analysis of serial sections (H and E, original magnification ×16). B. Detail of the cyst cavity. The lumen is filled with necrotic cells and tissue debris and infiltrated by many inflammatory cells (H and E, original magnification ×50). C. Magnification of the cyst wall in the area indicated by the arrow in B. Acute and chronic inflammatory cells in the epithelial lining and cyst lumen (H and E, original magnification ×400). D. High magnification of C (H and E, original magnification ×1000).

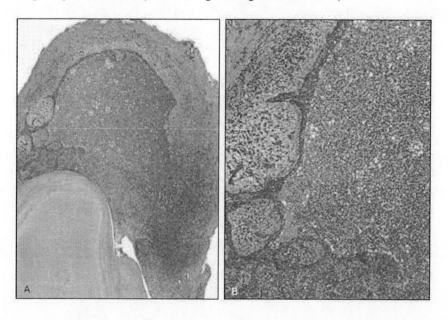

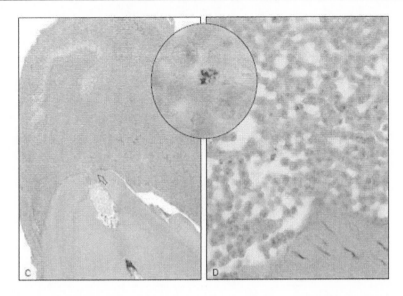

Figure 6. Extracted palatal root of a maxillary first molar with periapical lesion attached. In this section, not passing through the canal, the central part of the cystic apical periodontitis lesion is occupied by a large cavity lined by epithelium with no apparent communication with the root tip, which appears to be a true cyst (H and E, original magnification ×16). B. Detail of the left cyst wall and a part of lumen. There are several microabscesses in the epithelial lining and the lumen contains a dense concentration of PMNs, and (Hand E, original magnification ×50). C. Section taken approximately 100 after that shown in A, passing through the main foramen. Contrary to what appears in A, the cyst lumen is in communication with the root canal; therefore it is a "pocket cyst" (Taylor's modified Brown and Brenn, original magnification x16). D. Magnification of the area of the cyst lumen just beyond the apical foramen indicated by the arrow in C. Dense concentration of neutrophilic leukocytes, some of which show bacteria phagocytosed in their cytoplasm (Taylor's modified Brown and Brenn, original magnification × 400). Inset. Bacteria engulfed in the cytoplasm of a neutrophilic leukocyte (Taylor's modified Brown and Brenn, original magnification ×1000).

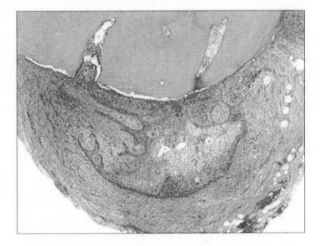

Figure 7. A radicular cyst formed at the apex of a tooth with complex apical anatomy. In this section, as well as in the neighbouring sections, it is not possible to establish whether there is a communication between the lumen of cyst and apical canal ramifications (H and E, original magnification ×25). Reprinted with permission from: Ricucci D. Patologia e Clinica. Endodontica. Edizioni Martina, Bologna, Italy, 2009.

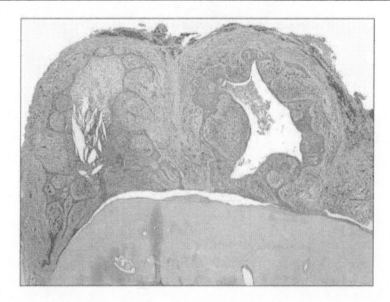

Figure 8. Two distinct cysts, separated by a fibrous connective tissue capsule, are present in the same apical periodontitis lesion at the apex of a maxillary second premolar (H and E, original magnification ×16).

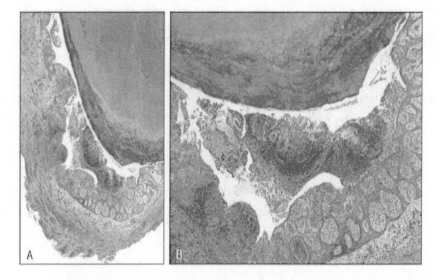

Figure 9. A. Apical periodontitis lesion at the periapex of a mandibular first premolar. A thick and arcaded epithelial lining exhibiting extensive proliferation surrounds a cavity containing debris. Serial sections demonstrate that this lesion is a pocket cyst (Masson trichrome, original magnification ×25). B. Detail of the cavity. Note many cyst-like cavities in proliferating epithelial lining (Masson trichrome, original magnification ×50).

epithelial lining exhibit extensive proliferation and may form an arcaded structure [Figure 9]. In inactive infection/inflammation, the epithelial lining is thin and regular and has minimal infiltration of inflammatory cells. Sometimes, ciliated or mucous cells may be seen in the epithelial lining of radicular cysts [Ricucci et al. 2006, Neville et al. 2009] [Figure 10].

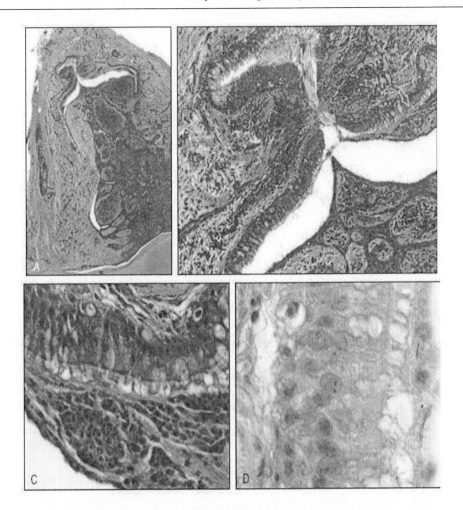

Figure 10. A. Cystic lesion at the periapex of the palatal root of a maxillary first molar (Hand E, original magnification ×25). B. Detail of the upper part of the lesion in A (H and E, original magnification ×100). C. Magnification of the area of the cyst wall indicated by the arrow in B. The epithelial lining consists of mucous producing ciliated columnar epithelial cells (goblet cells). The cyst cavity is occupied by a dense concentration of PMNs (H and E, original magnification ×400). D. High power view of the cyst wall. A pseudostratified ciliated columnar epithelium. Neutrophilic leukocytes can be seen in the cyst lumen (on the right) with some bacterial fragments in their cytoplasm (Taylor's modified Brown and Brenn, original magnification ×1000).

Often, Rushton bodies, presumably caused by hyaline degenerative changes in the walls of blood vessels, as eosinophilic, straight or curved, irregular or round structures are present within the epithelial lining of radicular cysts [Rushton 1955, Dunlap and Barker 1977] [Figure 11]. Occasionally, hyaline bodies, presumably caused by implantation of foreign food particles, can also be seen in the fibrous connective tissue capsule of radicular cysts [Talacko and Radden 1988, Chen et al. 1981]. The epithelial lining of cysts is separated from the underlying connective tissue by a basement membrane. Inflammatory cells usually infiltrate both epithelial lining and fibrous connective tissue capsule of the cysts [Figs. 3-10]. The lumen of cysts may contain necrotic tissue debris, dead or dying cells, lipid-filled foamy macrophages, and clear fluid [Figs. 3-10].

Cholesterol crystals associated with multinucleated giant cells may be seen in the fibrous connective tissue capsule and/or in the lumen of cysts [Lin et al. 2009] [Figure 8]. Bacteria have been observed in the lumen of radicular cysts [Ricucci et al. 2006].

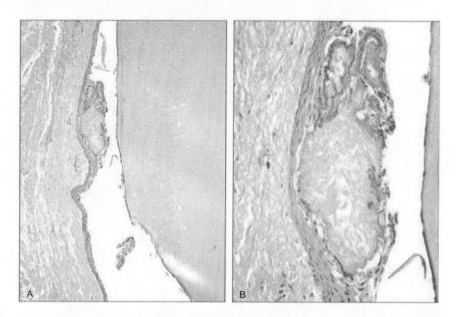

Figure 11. A. Stratified squamous epithelium lining a cyst at the apex of a mandibular second premolar exhibits irregular hyaline structures known as Rushton bodies (Taylor's modified Brown and Brenn, original magnification ×100). B. Magnification of the irregular body in A. A mass of necrotic debris surrounded by a fuchsine stained laminated structure, which appears circular or polycyclic on top (Taylor's modified Brown and Brenn, original magnification ×400).

DIAGNOSIS

Radicular cysts can only develop in an area of apical periodontitis. Therefore, the teeth involved usually have carious involvement, or a history of injury caused by trauma, or operative procedures. They do not respond to pulp tests with cold, heat, or electric pulp tester and are not sensitive to percussion and/or palpation. Residual cysts are not associated with cariously involved teeth or traumatized infected necrotic teeth. It is important to take a thorough dental history of teeth in the area of a possible residual cyst.

Conventional radiography, computed tomography, magnetic resonance imaging, and ultrasound may be able to detect changes at tissue or organ levels but not at a cellular level. They are used clinically to make a provisional clinical diagnosis of a disease entity or anomalies, which must be confirmed by histological examination. It is believed that if a periapical radiolucency is in excess of 2 cm^2, there is a strong probability that it may be cystic in nature [Lolonde 1970, Natkin et al. 1984] [Figure 12A]. In addition, a radicular cyst usually shows a well-localized periapical radiolucency bordered by a thin rim of cortical bone [Weber 1993, Scholl et al. 1999] [Figure .12B].

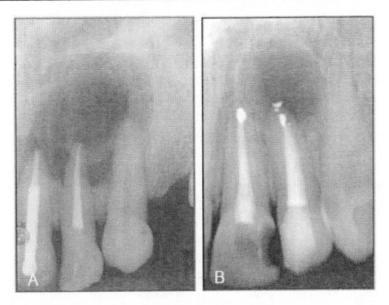

Figure 12. A-B. Large and corticated lesions are believed to be cystic in nature.

However, histological findings of periapical lesions showed poor correlation between the presence of a radiopaque lamina dura and a histological diagnosis of radicular cysts [Linenberg et al. 1964, Bhaskar 1966, Ricucci et al. 2006]. A study demonstrated that there was a high degree of correlation between the clinical radiographic diagnosis and the histological diagnosis of inflammatory radicular cysts [Lia et al. 2004]. In contrast, other studies have showed that it was difficult to diagnose radicular cysts based on radiographic findings [Priebe et al. 1954, Bhaskar 1966, Huumonen and Orstavik 2002].

Computed tomography has been shown to be superior to conventional radiography in detecting apical periodontitis [Cotti et al. 1999, Lofthan-Hansen et al. 2007, Estrela et al. 2008]. Several studies have demonstrated that computed tomography could differentiate radicular cysts from periapical granulomas [Trope et al. 1989, Simon et al. 2006, Cotton et al. 2007, Aggarwal et al. 2008]. However, a well-designed study involving multiple radiologists and pathologists showed that cone beam computed tomography was not a reliable diagnostic method for differentiating radicular cysts from periapical granulomas when compared to biopsy analysis [Rosenberg et al. 2010].

Magnetic resonance imaging [MRI] has been widely used in medicine but not in dentistry. MRI has been applied to detect dentigerous cysts [Gahleitner et al. 1999] and odontogenic keratocysts [Minami et al. 1996]. Ultrasound real time imaging has also been utilized to detect periapical bone lesions [Cotti et al. 2002]. Aggarwal et al. [2008] using ultrasound and histopathological diagnosis demonstrated that periapical granulomas could be differentiated from apical cysts by ultrasound with power Doppler flowmetry. Regardless of the diagnosis made by radiography, computed tomography, magnetic resonance imaging, or ultrasound, it must be confirmed by histological examination to arrive at a final diagnosis. The definitive, final diagnosis of radicular cysts can only be made through histological examination [Nair 1998].

REGRESSION OF RADICULAR CYSTS

Bhaskar [1972] examined 969 radicular cysts, which were excised for periods up to 8 months after the beginning of root canal therapy. He found that the epithelial lining of cysts was frequently infiltrated with polymorphonuclear leukocytes and was undergoing liquefaction, vacuolization, and disintegration. Therefore, he postulated that radicular cysts might undergo resolution after non-surgical root canal therapy if the root canal was instrumented slightly beyond the apex. As a result of this procedure, an acute inflammatory reaction might be induced and the epithelium of the cyst would be phagocytosed by polymorphonuclear leukocytes. Nevertheless, the epithelial lining of radicular cysts is usually infiltrated with polymorphonuclear leukocytes [Langeland et al. 1977, Nair et al. 1996, Ricucci et al. 2006]. Accordingly, it is not necessary to induce acute inflammation in cystic apical periodontitis lesions. In addition, it has not been demonstrated that polymorphonuclear leukocytes are capable of digesting epithelial cells [Seltzer 1988].

Torabinejad [1983] theorized that activated epithelial cell rests could acquire antigenic properties through ingestion of antigenic materials, which continuously egress from an infected necrotic root canal into the periapical tissues because epithelial cells are capable of phagocytosing foreign materials. The ingested material(s) and epithelial cells could be recognized as an antigenic unit. The activated epithelium could be destroyed by an antibody-dependent complement-mediated immune mechanism or cell-mediated immune mechanism through activated macrophages, cytotoxic T cells, or natural killer cells after root canal therapy. Apoptosis or programmed cell death is commonly seen in situations in which target cell destruction is induced by a cell-mediated immune response [Abbas et al. 2007]. Cytotoxic T cells, one of the effector cells of a cell-mediated immune response, can induce target cells to undergo apoptosis by two processes [Alberts et al. 2007]. In one process, cytotoxic T cells are activated by recognition of specific foreign antigens associated with MHC-1 on a target cell, they release perforin proteins that integrate into the membrane of the target cell and organize to form a membrane pore. This allows the protease granzyme to enter the cell and activate the apoptotic caspase proteolytic cascade [Alberts 2007]. The second process involves interaction of a cytotoxic T cell Fas ligand with the Fas receptor in the target cell. This activates the apoptotic caspase cascade [Alberts et al. 2007].

The biological nature of epithelial cells in proliferating epithelial strands or islands is similar to that of epithelial cells in radicular cysts in an area of apical periodontitis, because the epithelial cells are all derived from epithelial cell rests of Malassez [Lin et al. 2007]. From the outcome of non-surgical root canal therapy of teeth with apical periodontitis, approximately 52% of proliferated epithelial strands in apical periodontitis appear to be able to regress after periapical wound healing. Otherwise, a high percentage of teeth with apical periodontitis would show incompletely radiographic periapical wound healing after non-surgical root canal therapy. Therefore, if proliferated epithelial strands in an apical periodontitis are able to regress after non-surgical root canal therapy, the epithelial cells in radicular cysts should also be able to regress after non-surgical therapy. It was suggested based on cellular and molecular biology that inflammatory radicular cysts could regress after non-surgical root canal therapy, possibly by the mechanism of apoptosis/programmed cell death [Lin et al. 2007]. Apoptosis plays an important role in repair and regeneration of damaged tissue during wound healing [Greenhalgh 1998, Rai et al. 2005]. Cells not originally present in the injured tissue, such as inflammatory cells and excess cells, for example, endothelial cells, fibroblasts, and epithelial cells are eliminated during wound healing and restore the original tissue architecture [Greenhalgh 1998, Rai et al. 2005]. Dysregulation of apoptosis can result in abnormal wound healing [Desmouliere et al. 1997, Jones and Gores 1997].

After non-surgical root canal therapy, the basal stem cells of the epithelial lining of inflammatory radicular cysts stop proliferating because of a reduction in inflammatory mediators, pro-inflammatory cytokines, and growth factors. As periapical wound healing progresses, epithelial cells of inflammatory cysts are deprived of survival/growth factors and their apoptotic signal is activated [Collins et al. 1994, Jilka et al. 1998, Bergmann 2002, Letai 2006, Lodish et al. 2007]. A reduction or deprivation of inflammatory mediators, pro-inflammatory cytokines, and growth factors has been shown to result in regression of inflammatory hyperplastic epithelium in several epithelial tissues, such as liver [Bursch et al. 1985], kidney [Ledda-Columbano et al. 1989], larynx [Hellquist 1997], and gallbladder [Bhathal and Gall 1985]. It is well known that *H. pylori* infection is commonly seen associated with hyperplastic polyps of the stomach. Hyperplastic polyps can regress through apoptosis after early elimination of *H. pylori* [Ohkusa et al. 1998, Nakajima et al. 2000].

Loyola et al. [2005], using antibody against pro-apoptotic factor, Bcl-2 antigen, showed that apoptosis was observed in both hyperplastic and atrophic epithelial linings of apical cysts. Suzuki et al. [2005] demonstrated that apoptotic cell death occurred in the epithelial lining of apical and residual apical cysts by using monoclonal antibodies or polyclonal antisera against single-stranded DNA and P53, Bax, Bcl-2, caspase-3, Fas-L, or Ki-67 antigen. Martins et al. [2011] also showed that pro-apoptotic factor, caspase-3 was detected in the suprabasal and superficial epithelial cells and Bcl-2 was restricted to the basal layer of radicular cysts using immunohistochemical analysis.

It was postulated in one case report that inflammatory true cysts are less likely to regress after non-surgical root canal therapy because they are no longer dependent on the presence or absence of irritants in the root canal. Therefore inflammatory true cysts are self-sustaining [Nair 1998]. Biologically, no studies have demonstrated that inflammatory pocket cysts are different from inflammatory true cysts [Ricucci et al. 2006]. Both pocket and true apical cysts are formed in an area of apical periodontitis and derived from epithelial cell rests. Consequently, similar to pocket cysts, inflammatory true cysts have the potential to regress following non-surgical root canal therapy, possibly by the mechanism of apoptosis [Lin et al. 2009]. If inflammatory apical true cysts were self-sustaining, it would indicate that they were neoplastic. No evidence has indicated that an inflammatory apical true cyst is a neoplastic lesion. It must be emphasized that failure of treatment of cystic apical periodontitis is due to persistent intraradicular infection or reinfection of the canal of involved teeth [Siqueira et al. 2001, Ricucci et al. 2009].

Cholesterol crystals, a product of apical periodontitis, have also been suggested as a possible factor preventing healing of apical periodontitis lesions, especially in inflammatory apical true cysts, after non-surgical root canal therapy [Nair et al. 1993, Nair et al. 1998, Nair 1999]. The incidence of cholesterol crystals present in apical periodontitis lesions (granulomas and cysts) has been estimated to range from 12 to 44% [Shears 1963, Trott et al. 1973, Bhaskar 1966, Browne 1971, Iqbal 2008]. If cholesterol crystals alone could prevent periapical wound healing, then 12 to 44% of apical periodontitis lesions containing cholesterol crystals would not heal after non-surgical root canal therapy. This is not consistent

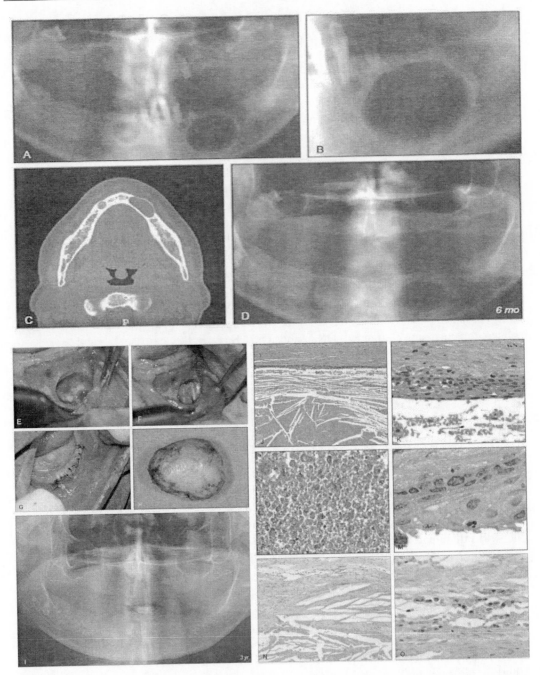

Figure 13. A. Panoramic radiograph of a 55-yr-old woman. Several large radiolucent lesions are present in maxilla and mandible, likely to be of endodontic origin. B. Detail of the radiograph showing that the large radiolucent lesion on the left mandible is associated with a residual root. C. Computed tomography showing the extent of the large radiolucent lesion in B. D. A new panoramic radiograph taken 6 months after extraction of all teeth showed that the large periapical radiolucent lesion on the left mandible remained almost the same size, while all other periapical radiolucent lesions resolved completely. E-G. It was decided to surgically enucleate the large residual periapical radiolucent lesion on the left mandible and to perform histologic examination. H. Specimen of a lesion enucleated from E. I. A follow-up panoramic radiograph taken 3 years after surgical intervention showing that the radiolucent lesion has been filled by newly formed bone. J. Low magnification of the cyst wall and

lumen. Thin stratified squamous epithelium surrounding a cavity filled with necrotic debris and blood cells. Numerous empty spaces in the lumen, indicative of cholesterol crystals dissolved during histological processing (H and E, original magnification ×50). K. Detail of the cyst wall. Thin epithelial lining infiltrated with minimal inflammatory cells (H and E, original magnification ×400). L. High power view from the center of the cavity, showing necrotic debris and no viable cells at this level (H and E, original magnification ×400). M. At high magnification, one neutrophilic leukocyte close to the cyst lumen transmigrating through the epithelial lining (H and E, original magnification ×1000). N. In some areas, cholesterol crystals can be seen in the fibrous connective tissue wall of the cyst. Bacteria are absent (Taylor's modified Brown and Brenn staining, original magnification ×100). O. High magnification of the upper portion of the cyst wall in N. Mild infiltration of chronic inflammatory cells. Bacteria are absent (Taylor's modified Brown and Brenn staining, original magnification ×400). This case is the courtesy of Dr. Luigi Occhiuzzi, Cetraro, Italy.

with well-conducted long-term outcome studies of endodontically involved teeth with apical periodontitis after non-surgical root canal therapy. If negative bacterial cultures are obtained and root canal fillings are 0-2 mm from the radiographic apex, the success rate of non-surgical root canal therapy of teeth with apical periodontitis is approximately 94%, regardless of whether cholesterol crystals are present or not in the inflammatory periapical lesions [Sjögren et al. 1990, Sjögren et al. 1997]. However, cholesterol crystals may delay wound healing of apical periodontitis lesions after non-surgical root canal therapy.

Residual cysts are not associated with infected necrotic teeth (Figure 13). The irritants sustaining persistence of inflammatory residual cysts are likely to be around or in the cyst itself. Therefore, a decompression procedure or a surgical intervention may be a treatment possibility and will be discussed in the following section. Oehlers [1970] observed that many inflammatory residual cysts regressed after extraction of the involved teeth. The residual epithelial lining underwent atrophy because the factors responsible for cystic growth had been removed. On occasion, inflammatory residual cysts show spontaneous regression if inflammation is not a prominent feature [Oehlers 1970, High and Hirschmann 1986].

A frequently asked question is "can radicular cysts recur if their epithelial lining is not completely removed during periapical surgery?" This has been previously discussed [Lin et al. 1996]. The epithelial cells of epithelial linings of radicular cysts are not neoplastic cells. Similar to proliferated epithelial strands or islands in an area of apical periodontitis after non-surgical root canal therapy, the incompletely removed epithelial linings after surgery have the potential to regress, possibly by the mechanism of apoptosis. However, this only occurs in the absence of infection/inflammation in the root canal system or in the periapical tissues.

TREATMENT OPTIONS

Since radicular cysts cannot be diagnosed clinically with certainty before treatment, controversy continues whether radicular cysts can or cannot be treated with non-surgical endodontic therapy. Some clinicians [Patterson et al. 1964] believe that inflammatory radicular cysts, like all other non-inflammatory odontogenic and non-odontogenic cysts, require surgical enucleation without providing any reasonable biological explanation. There are no cysts in the human body, which are formed in a similar process to a radicular cyst, by inflammatory proliferation of epithelial cell rests in an area of apical periodontitis. Inflammatory radicular cysts are not developmental or neoplastic cysts, which require surgical intervention to remove the lesions.

As previously mentioned, radicular cysts cannot be diagnosed clinically before treatment and there is the potential for radicular cysts to regress by the mechanism of apoptosis after control of root canal infection. Therefore, all cyst-like inflammatory periapical lesions associated with endodontically involved teeth should be initially treated by non-surgical endodontic therapy. Clinical prognosis studies of large cyst-like inflammatory periapical lesions following complete nonsurgical root canal treatment have showed favorable results [Bhaskar 1972, Çalışkan 2004, Soares et al. 2006, Fernandes and de Ataide 2010, Venugopal et al. 2011]. No studies or case reports have convincingly demonstrated that surgical removal of inflammatory radicular cysts (true and pocket) without effective control of root canal infection, such as root resection in conjunction with complete root-end filling could predictably result in healing of cystic apical periodontitis.

Decompression procedures followed by non-surgical root canal therapy have also been recommended to treat large cyst-like inflammatory periapical lesions, which may involve the maxillary sinus, mental foramen, or mandibular canal [Neaverth and Burg 1982, Loushine et al. 1991, Rees 1997, Oztan 2002, Martin 2007, Fernandes and de Ataide 2010, Tandri 2010]. The decompression procedures involve placement of a drain into the cystic lesion, regular irrigation, adjustment and maintenance of the drain, for various periods of time [Loushine et al. 1991]. The purpose of decompression procedures is to reduce the size of cystic lesions. The patient's cooperation is important in decompression procedures. If surgical treatment of large cyst-like inflammatory periapical lesions is a slected as the treatment option, care must be taken to avoid injury to adjacent vital teeth and adjacent vital structures. However, a combination of an initial decompression procedure to reduce the size of large cyst-like lesions, followed by a surgical procedure may be a better choice to prevent damage to adjacent vital teeth and adjacent vital structures than surgery alone [Torres-Lagareset al. 2011]. Residual cysts can be treated surgically and result in satisfactory healing (Figure 13).

What are the differences between non-surgical and surgical treatment of radicular cysts? During surgical endodontic treatment, a clinician attempts to remove the radicular cyst in total or, at least, most of the cyst. Therefore, fresh fibrovascular granulation tissue grows immediately into the surgically debrided area to initiate wound healing. In non-surgical endodontic treatment, activated macrophages perform phagocytosis of necrotic cells, tissue debris and apoptotic epithelial cells of radicular cyst in the periapical area. Accordingly, fresh fibrovascular granulation tissue grows slowly into the periapical wound as activated macrophages gradually remove necrotic cells and tissue to initiate wound healing. Therefore, considering the short-term outcome, surgical endodontic therapy of radicular cysts heals more rapidly than non-surgical endodontic therapy [Kvist and Reit 1999]. However, the long-term outcome of surgical and non-surgical endodontic therapy of cyst-like periapical lesions is the same [Kvist and Reit 1999]. The principle of treatment of diseases caused by infection is to control infection [Mims et al. 2004]. Again, simply removing inflammatory radicular cysts [pocket and true] without effective control of root canal infection will not result in healing of cystic apical periodontitis. It is important to note that surgical biopsy specimens must be sent for histopathologic examination to confirm the clinical diagnosis.

CONCLUSION

Radicular and residual cysts are the product of apical periodontitis caused by root canal infection. They are not developmental or neoplastic cysts. As in other infectious diseases, radicular cysts have the potential to regress, possibly by the mechanism of apoptosis, after control of infection by conservative non-surgical root canal therapy.

REFERENCES

Abbas AK, Lichtman AH, Pillai S. Cellular and Molecular Immunology. 6th ed. Philadelphia: Saunders 2007.

Aggarwal V, Logani A, Shah N. The evaluation of computed tomography scans and ultrasounds in differential diagnosis of periapical lesions. *J. Endod.* 2008; 34: 1312-5.

Alberts B, Bray D, Lewis J, et al. Molecular Biology of the Cell. 4th ed. New York: Garland Publishing, Inc. 2007.

Barnes L, Everson JW, Reichart PA, et al. Pathology and genetics of head and heck tumor. World Health Organization classification of tumors. Lyon, France: IARC Press 2005.

Barreto DC, Gomez RS, Bale AE, et al. PTCH gene mutations in odontogenic keratocysts. *J. Dent. Res.* 2000; 79: 1418-22.

Bergmann A. Survival signaling goes BAD. *Dev. Cell* 2002; 3: 607-8.

Berstad AE, Hatlebakk JG, Maartmann-Moe H, et al. *Helicobacter pylori* and epithelial cell proliferation in patients with reflux esophagitis after treatment with lansoprazole. *Gut* 1997; 41: 740-747.

Bhaskar SN. Oral pathology in the dental office: survey of 20,575 biopsy specimens. *J. Am. Dent. Assoc.* 1968; 76: 761-6.

Bhaskar S. Nonsurgical resolution of radicular cysts. *Oral. Surg.* 1972; 34: 458-68.

Bhaskar SN. Periapical lesions – Types, incidence and clinical features. *Oral. Surg. Oral. Med. Oral. Pathol.* 1966; 21: 657-71.

Bhathal PS, Gall JAM. Deletion of hyperplastic biliary epithelial cells by apoptosis following removal of the proliferative stimulus. *Liver* 1985; 5: 311-25.

Block RM, Bushell A, Rodrigues H, Langeland K. A histologic, histobacteriologic, and radiographic study of periapical endodontic surgical specimens. *Oral. Surg. Oral. Med. Oral. Pathol.* 1976; 42: 656-78.

Browne RM. The origin of cholesterol in odontogenic cysts in man. *Arch. Oral. Biol.* 1971; 16: 107-13.

Brunette DM. Cholera toxin and dibutyl cyclic-AMP stimulate the growth of epithelial cells derived from epithelial cell rests from porcine periodontal ligament. *Arch. Oral. Biol.* 1984; 39: 303-9.

Bursch W, Taper HS, Lauer B, Schulte-Hermann R. Quantitative histological and histochemical studies on the occurrence and stage of controlled cell death (apoptosis) during regression of rat liver hyperplasia. *Virchows Arch. B. Cell Pathol. Uncl. Mol. Pathol.* 1985; 50: 153-66.

Çalışkan MK. Prognosis of large cyst-like periapical lesions following nonsurgical root canal treatment: a clinical review. *Int. Endod. J.* 2004; 37: 408-16.

Chedid M, Rubin JS, Csaky KG. Regulation of keratinocyte growth factor expression by interleukin 1. *J. Biol. Chem.* 1994; 269: 10753-7.

Chang K-M, Lehrhaupt N, Lin LM, Feng J, Wu-Wang C-Y, Wang S-L. Epidermal growth factor in gingival crevicular fluid and its binding capacity in inflamed and non-inflamed human gingival, *Arch. Oral. Biol.* 1996; 41: 719-34.

Chen S, Fantasia JE, Miller AS. Hyaline bodies in connective tissue wall of odontogenic cysts. *J. Oral. Pathol.* 1981; 10: 147-57.

Colic M, Gazivoda D, Vucevic D, et al. Proinflammatory and immunoregulatory mechanisms in periapical lesions. *Mol. Immunol.* 2009; 47: 101-13.

Collins ANP, Lomago BL, Swalsky AD, et al. Molecular analysis to demonstrate that odontogenic keratocysts are neoplastic. *Arch. Pathol. Lab. Med.* 2004; 128: 313-7.

Collins MKL, Perkins GR, Rodriguez-Tarduchy G, Nieto MA, Lopez-Rivas Growth factors as survival factors: Regulation of apoptosis. *BioEssays* 1994; 16: 133-8.

Cotti E, Campisi G, Garau V, Puddu G. A new technique for the study of periapical bone lesions. *Int. Endod. J.* 2002; 35: 148-52.

Cotti E, Vargiu P. Dettori C, Mallarini G. Computerized tomography in the treatment and follow-up of extensive periapical lesion. *Endod. Dent. Traumatol.* 1999; 15: 186-9.

Cotton TP, Geisler TM, Holden DT, et al. Endodontic applications of cone- beam volumetric tomography. *J. Endod.* 2007; 33: 1121-32.

Desmouliere A, Badid C, Bochaon-Piallat M-L, Gabbiani G. Apoptosis during wound healing, fibrocontractive diseases and vascular wall injury. *Int. J. Biochem. Cell Biol.* 1997; 29: 19-30.

Dunlap CL, Barker BF. Giant-cell hyaline angiopathy. *Oral. Surg. Oral. Med. Oral. Pathol.* 1977; 44: 587-91.

Estrela C, Bueno MR, Leles CR, et al. Accuracy of cone beam computed tomography and panoramic and periapical radiography for detection of apical periodontitis. *J. Endod.* 2008; 34: 273-9.

Femiano F, Lanza A, Buonaiuto C, et al. Pyostomatitis vegetans: A review of literature. *Med. Oral. Pathol. Oral. Cir. Buccal.* 2009; 14: E114-7.

Fernandes M, de Ataide I. Nonsurgical management of periapical lesions. *J. Conserv. Dent.* 2010; 13: 240-5.

Fouad AF. IL-1*a* and TNF-*a* expression in early periapical lesions of normal and immunodeficient mice. *J. Dent. Res.* 1997; 76: 1548-54.

Gao Z, FlaitzCM, Mackenzie IC. Expression of keratinocyte growth factor in periapical lesions. *J. Dent. Res.* 1996; 75: 1658-663.

Gahleitner A, Solar P, Nasel C, et al. Magnetic resonance tomography and dental radiology (Dental-MRT). *Radiology* 1999; 39: 1044-50.

Greenhalgh DG. The role of apoptosis in wound healing. *Int. J. Biochem Cell Biol.* 1998; 30: 1019-30.

Grossman RM, Kreuger J, Yourish A, et al. Interleukin-6 is expressed in high levels in psoriatic skin and stimulates proliferation of cultured human keratinocytes. *Proc. Nat. Acad. Sci. USA* 1989; 86: 6367-71.

Haegens A, van der Vllet A, Butnor KJ, et al. Asbestos-induced lung inflammation and epithelial cell proliferation are altered in myeloperoxidase-null mice. *Cancer Res.* 2005; 65: 9670-9777.

Hahn C-L, Liewebr FR. Innate immune responses of the dental pulp to caries. *J. Endod.* 2007a; 33: 643-51.

Hahn C-L, Liewebr FR. Update on the adaptive immune responses of the dental pulp. *J. Endod.* 2007b; 33: 773-81.

Hellquist HB. Apoptosis in epithelial hyperplastic laryngeal lesions. *Acta Otolaryngol.* 1997; 117: 25-9.

Heyeraas KJ, Berggreen E. Interstitial fluid pressure in normal and inflamed pulp. *Crit. Rev. Oral. Biol. Med.* 1999; 10: 328-36.

High AS, Hirschmann PN. Age changes in residual radicular cysts. *J. Oral. Pathol. Med.* 1986; 15: 524-528.

Huumonen S, Ørstavik D. Radiological aspects of apical periodontitis. *Endod. Topics* 2002; 1: 3-25.

Ihan HN, Ihan A. T lymphocyte activation and cytokine expression in periapical granulomas and radicular cysts. *Arch. Oral. Biol.* 2009; 54: 156-61.

Iqbal MF. The relationship between cholesterol crystals, foamy macrophages, and hemosiderine in odontogenic cysts. A treatise for the degree of Masters in Dental Science. Department of Oral Medicine and Oral Pathology, Faculty of Dentistry, The University of Sydney, Australia 2008.

Irwin CR, Schor SL Ferguson MW. Expression of EGF-receptor on epithelial and stromal cells of normal and inflamed gingival. *J. Periodont. Res.* 1991; 26: 388-94.

Jilka RL, Weinstein RS, Bellido T, et al. Osteoblast programmed cell death (Apoptosis): Modulation by growth factors and cytokines. *J. Bone Miner Res.* 1998; 13: 793-802.

Jones BA, Gores GJ. Physiology and pathophysiology of apoptosis in epithelial cells of the liver, pancreas, and intestine. *Am. J. Physiol. Gastrointest. Liver Physiol.* 1997; 273; G1174-88.

Kakehashi S, Stanley HR, Fitzgerald RJ. The effects of surgical exposures of dental pulps in germ-free and conventional laboratory rats. *Oral. Surg. Oral. Med. Oral. Pathol.* 1965; 20: 340-9.

Kawashima N, Stashenko P. Expression of bone-resorptive and regulatory cytokines in murine periapical inflammation. *Arch. Oral. Biol.* 1999; 44: 55.

Keutteke NC, Lee DC. Transforming growth factor alpha: expression, regulation and biological action of its integral membrane precursor EGF family of receptors and ligands. 1. Structure and function. In: Dickerson RB, Lippmann ME, eds. Seminar in Cancer Biology. Vol 1. Philadelphia: Saunders 1990: 265-75.

Koseoglu BG, Atalay B, Erdem MA. Odontogenic cysts: a clinical study of 90 cases. *J. Oral. Sci.* 2004; 46: 253-7.

Kovacevic M, Tamarut T, Jonjic N, et al. The transition from pulpitis to periapical periodontitis in dog's teeth. *Aust. Endod. J.* 2008; 34: 12-8.

Kramer IR, Pindborg JJ, Shear M. The WHO Histological Typing of Odontogenic Tumors: a commentary on the second edition. *Cancer* 1992; 70: 2988-94.

Kvist T, Reit C. Results of endodontic retreatment: a randomized clinical study comparing surgical and non-surgical procedures. *J. Endod.* 1999; 25: 220-7.

Kumar V, Abbas AK, Fausto N, et al. Pathologic Basis of Disease. 8th ed. Philadelphia: Saunders 2009.

Lalonde ER. A new rationale for the management of periapical granulomas and cysts: a an evaluation of histopathological and radiographic findings. *J. Am. Dent. Assoc.* 1970; 80: 1056-9.

Langeland K, Block RM, Grossman LI. A histopathologic study of 35 periapical endodontic surgical specimens. *J. Endod.* 1977; 3: 8-23.

Ledda-Columbano GM, Columbano A, Coni P, et al. Cell deletion by apoptosis during regression of renal hyperplasia. *Am. J. Pathol.* 1989; 135: 657-62.

Letai A. Growth factor withdrawal and apoptosis: The middle game. *Mol. Cell.* 2006; 21: 728-730.

Li TJ, Browne RM, Mathews JB. Expression of epidermal growth factor receptors by odontogenic jaw cysts. *Virchows* 1993; 423: 137-44.

Li, T-J. The odontogenic keratocyst: A cyst, or a cystic neoplasm? *J. Dent. Res.* 2011; 90: 133-42.

Lia RCC, Garcia JMQ, Sousa-Neto MD, et al. Clinical, radiographic and histological evaluation of chronic periapical inflammatory lesions. *J. Applied Oral. Sci.* 2004; 12: 117-20.

Lin LM, Gaegler P, Langeland K. Periapical curettage. *Int. Endod. J.* 1996; 29; 220-7.

Lin LM, Wang SL, Wu-Wang C, et al. Detection of epidermal growth factor receptor in inflammatory periapical lesions. *Int. Endod. J.* 1996; 29: 179-84.

Lin LM, Pascon EA, Skribner J, et al. Clinical, radiographic, and histological study of endodontic treatment failures. *Oral. Surg. Oral. Med. Oral. Pathol.* 1991; 71: 603-11.

Lin LM, Ricucci D, Lin J, Rosenberg PA. Nonsurgical root canal therapy of large cyst-like inflammatory periapical lesions an inflammatory apical cysts. *J. Endod.* 2009; 35: 607-15.

Lin LM, Huang G T-J, Rosenberg PA. Proliferation of epithelial cell rests, formation of apical cysts, and regression of apical cysts after periapical wound healing. *J. Endod.* 2007; 33: 908-16.

Linenberg WB, Waldron CA, DeLaune GF. A clinical, roentgenographic, and histopathologic evaluation of periapical lesions. *Oral. Surg. Oral. Med. Oral. Pathol.* 1964; 17: 467-72.

Lodish H, Berk A, Matsudaira P, et al. Molecular Cell Biology. New York: WH Freeman 2007.

Lofthang-Hansen S, Huumonen S, Grondahl K, Grondahl H-G. Limited cone-beam CT and intraoral radiography for the diagnosis of periapical pathology. *Oral. Surg. Oral. Med. Oral. Pathol. Oral. Radiol. Endod.* 2007; 103: 114-9.

Loushine RJ, Weller RN, Bellizzi R, Kulild JC. A 2-day decompression: A case report of a maxillary first molar. *J. Endod.* 1991; 17: 85-7.

Love RM, Firth N, Histopathological profile of surgically removed persistent periapical radiolucent lesions of endodontic origin. *Int. Endo J* 2009; 42: 198-202.

Loyola AM, Cardoso SV, Lisa GS, et al. Apoptosis in epithelial cells of apical radicular cysts. *Int. Endod. J.* 2005; 38: 465-9.

MacDonald TT. Epithelial proliferation in response to gastrointestinal inflammation. *Ann. NY Acad. Sci.* 1992; 664: 202-209.

Main DMG. Epithelial jaw cysts. 10 years of WHO classification. *J. Oral. Pathol. Med* 1985; 14: 1-7.

Majno G, Joris I. Cells, Tissues, and Disease. 2nd ed. Oxford: Oxford University Press 2004.

Marcal JRB, Samuel RO, Fernandes D, et al. T-helper cell type 17/regulatory T-cell immunoregulatory balance in human radicular cysts and periapical granulomas. *J. Endod.* 2010; 36: 995-9.

Martin SA. Conventional endodontic therapy of upper central incisor combined with cyst decompression: A case report. *J. Endod.* 2007; 33: 753-7.

Martins CA, Rivero ERC, Dufloth RM, et al. Immunohistochemical detection of factors related to cellular proliferation and apoptosis in radicular cysts and dentigerous cysts. *J. Endod.* 2011; 37: 36-9.

McHugh WD, Zander HA. Cell division in the periodontium of developing and erupted teeth. *Dent. Pract. Dent. Rec.* 1965; 15: 451-7.

Meghji S, Qureshi W, Henderson B, Harris M. The role of endotoxin and cytokines in the pathogenesis of odontogenic cysts. *Arch. Oral. Biol.* 1996; 41: 523-31.

Mims C, Playfair J, Roitt I, et al. Medical Microbiology. 3rd ed. Philadelphia: Mosby 2004.

Minami M, Kaneda T, Ozawa K, et al. Cystic lesions of the maxillomandibular region: MR imaging distinction of odontogenic keratocysts and ameloblastomas from other cysts. *Am. J. Roentgenol.* 1996; 943-9.

Möller AJR, Fabricius L, Dahlén G, Ohman AE, Heyden G. Influence of periapical tissues of indigenous oral bacteria and necrotic pulp tissue in monkeys. *Scand. J. Dent. Res.* 1981; 89: 475-84.

Mortensen H, Winter JE, Birn H. Periapical granulomas and cysts. *Scand. J. Dent. Res.* 1970; 78: 241-50.

Nakajima A, Matsuhashi N, Yazaki Y, et al. Details of hyperplastic polyps of the stomach shrinking after anti-Helicobacter pylori therapy. *J. Gastroenterol.* 2000; 35: 372-5.

Nakamura T, Ishida J, Nakano Y, et al. A study of cysts in the oral region. Cysts of the jaw. *J. Nihon Univ. Sch. Dent.* 1995; 37: 33-40.

Nanci A. Ten Cate's Oral Biology. 7th ed. St. Louis: Mosby 2007.

Nair PNR. New perspectives on radicular cysts: do they heal? *Int. Endod. J.* 1998; 31: 155-60.

Nair PNR. Cholesterol as an aetiological agent in endodontic failure: a review. *Aut. Endod. J.* 1999; 25: 19-26.

Nair PNR. Pathogenesis of apical periodontitis and the causes of endodontic failures. *Crit. Rev. Oral. Biol. Med.* 2004; 15: 348-81.

Nair PNR, Pajarola G, Schroeder HE. Types and incidence of human periapical lesions obtained with extracted teeth. *Oral. Surg. Oral. Med. Oral. Pathol.* 1996; 81: 93-102.

Nair PNR, Sjögren U, Schumacher E, Sundqvist G. Radicular cyst affecting a root filled human tooth: A long term post treatment follow-up. *Int. Endod. J.* 1993; 26: 225-300.

Nair PNR, Sjögren U, Sundqvist G. Cholesterol crystals as an etiologic factor in nonresolving chronic inflammation: an experimental study in guinea pigs. *Eur. J. Oral. Sci.* 1998; 106: 644-50.

Nair PNR, Sundqvist G, Sjögren U. Experimental evidence supports the abscess theory of development of radicular cysts. *Oral. Surg. Oral. Med. Oral. Pathol. Oral. Radiol. Endod.* 2008; 106: 294-303.

Natkin E, Oswald RJ, Carnes LL. The relationship of lesion size to diagnosis, incidence, and treatment of periapical cyst and granulomas. *Oral. Surg. Oral. Med. Oral. Pathol.* 1984; 57: 82-94.

Neaverth EJ, Burg HA. Decompression of large periapical cystic lesions. *J. Endod.* 1982; 8: 175-82.

Neville BW, Damm DD, Allen CM, Bouquot JE. Oral and Maxillofacial Pathology. 3rd ed. St. Louis: Saunders 2009.

Nobuhara WK, Del Rio CE. Incidence of periapical pathoses in endodontic treatment failures. *J. Endod.* 1993; 19: 315-8.

Nordlund L, Hormia M, Saxen L, Thesleff I. Immunohistochemical localization of epidermal growth factor receptors in human gingival epithelia. *J. Periodont. Res.* 1991; 26: 333-8.

Oehlers FAC. Periapical lesions and residual dental cysts. *Br. J. Oral. Surg.* 1970; 8: 103-13.

Ohkusa T, Takashimizu I, Fujiki K, et al. Disappearance of hyperplastic polyps in the stomach after eradication of *Heliobacter pylori*: a randomized, controlled trail. *Ann. Intern. Med.* 1998; 129: 712-5.

Oztan MD. Endodontic treatment of teeth associated with a large periapical lesion. *Int. Endod. J.* 2002; 35: 73-8.

Patterson SS, Shafer WG, Healey HG. Periapical lesions associated with endodontically treated teeth. *J. Am. Dent. Assoc.* 1964; 68: 191-4.

Priebe WA, Lazonsky JP, Wuehrman AH. Value of the roentgenographic film in the differential diagnosis of periapical lesions. *Oral. Surg. Oral. Med. Oral. Pathol.* 1954; 7: 979-83.

Rai NK, Tripathi K, Sharma D, et al. Apoptosis: A basic physiologic process in wound healing. *Lower Extremity Wiunds* 2005; 4: 138-44.

Rees JS. Conservative management of a large maxillary cyst. *Int. Endod. J.* 1997; 30: 64-7.

Reeves CM, Wentz FM. The prevalence, morphology, and distribution of epithelial rests in human periodontal ligament. *Oral. Surg.* 1962; 5: 254-8.

Ricciardolo FLM, Di Stefano A, van Krieken JHJM, et al. Proliferation and inflammation in bronchial epithelium after allergen in atopic asthmatics. *Clin. Exp. Allergy* 2003; 33: 905-911.

Ricucci D, Mannocci F, Pitt Ford TR. A study of periapical lesions correlating the presence of a radiopaque lamina with histological findings. *Oral. Surg. Oral. Med. Oral. Pathol. Oral. Radiol. Endod.* 2006a; 101: 389-94.

Ricucci D, Martorano M, Bate AL, Pascon EA. Calculs-like deposit on the apical external root surface of teeth with post-treatment apical periodontitis: report of two cases. *Int. Endo. J.* 2005; 38: 262-71.

Ricucci D, Pascon EA, Pitt Ford TR, Langeland K. Epithelium and bacteria in periapical lesions. *Oral. Surg. Oral. Med. Oral. Pathol. Oral. Radiol. Endod.* 2006b; 101: 239-49.

Ricucci D, Siqueira JF Jr, Bate AL, Pitt Ford TR. Histologic investigation of root canal with apical periodontitis: a retrospective study from 24 patients. *J. Endod.* 2009; 35: 493-502.

Ricucci D, Siqueira JF. Biofilm and apical periodontitis: study of prevalence and association with clinical and histological findings. *J. Endod.* 2010; 36: 1277-88.

Rosenberg PA, Frisbie J, Lee J, Lee K. et al. Evaluation of pathologists (histopathology) and radiologists (cone beam computed tomography) differentiating radicular cysts from granulomas. *J. Endod.* 2010; 36: 423-8.

Rushton MA. Hayline bodies in the epithelium of dental cysts. *Proc. Royal Soc. Med.* 1955; 48: 407-9.

Sanchis JM, Penarrocha M, Bagan JV, et al. Incidence of radicular cysts in a series of 125chronic periapical lesions. *Rev. Stomatol. Chir. Maxillofac.* 1998; 98: 354-8.

Sauder DN. Interleukin-1 in dermatological disease: In Bomford R, Henderson B, eds. Interleukin-1, Inflammation and Disease. North Holland: Elsevier 1989: 257.

Scholl RJ, Kellett HM, Neumann DP, Lurie AG. Cysts and cystic lesions of the mandible: clinical and radiographic-histopathologic review. *RadioGraphics* 1999; 19: 1107-24.

Schulz M, von Arx T, Altermatt HJ, et al. Histology of periapical lesions obtained during apical surgery. *J. Endod.* 2009; 35: 634-42.

Seltzer S, Bender LB, Smith J, et al. Endodontic failures – an analysis based on clinical, roentgenographic, and histologic findings. Part 1. *Oral. Surg. Oral. Med. Oral. Pathol.* 1967; 23: 500-16.

Seltzer S. Endodontology: Biological considerations in endodontic procedures. Philadelphia: Lea and Febiger 1988.

Seltzer S, Soltanoff W, Bender IB. Epithelial proliferation in periapical lesions. *Oral. Surg. Oral. Med. Oral. Pathol.* 1969; 27: 111-21.

Shankar N, Lockatell V, Baghdayan AS, et al. Role of *Enterococcus faecalis* surface protein Esp in the pathogenesis of ascending urinary tract infection. *Infect. Immun.* 2001; 69: 4366-72.

Shears M. The histogenesis of dental cysts. *Dent. Pract.* 1963; 13: 238-43.

Sjögren U, Figdor D, Persson S, Sundqvist G. Influence of infection at the time of root filling on the outcome of endodontic treatment of teeth with apical periodontitis. *Int. Endod. J.* 1997; 30: 297-306.

Sjögren U, Hägglund B, Sundqvist G, Wing K. Factors affecting the long-term results of endodontic treatment. *J. Endod.* 1990; 10: 498-503.

Simon JHS, Incidence of periapical cysts in relation to root canal. *J. Endod.* 1980; 76: 356-61.

Simon HHS, Enciso R, Malfaz J-M, et al. Differential diagnosis of large periapical lesions using cone-beam computed tomography measurements and biopsy. *J. Endod.* 2006; 32: 833-37.

Siqueira JF Jr. Aetiology of root canal treatment failure: Why well-treated teeth can fail. *Int. J. Endod.* 2001; 34: 1-10.

Soares J, Santos S, Silveira F, Nunes E. Nonsurgical treatment of extensive cyst-like periapical lesion of endodontic origin. *Int. J. Endod.* 2006; 39: 566-75.

Spatafore CM, Griffin JA, Keyes GG, et al. Periapical biopsy reports: an analysis of a 10-year period. *J. Endod.* 1990; 16: 239-41.

Stashenko P, Teles R, D'Souza R. Periapical inflammatory responses and their modulation. *Crit. Rev. Oral. Biol. Med.* 1998; 9: 498-521.

Stockdale CR, Chandler NP. The nature of periapical lesions – a review of 1108 cases. *J. Dent.* 1988; 16: 123-9.

Strohl WA, Rouse H, Fisher B, Harvey RA, Champe PC. Microbiology. Baltimore: Lippincott Williams and Wilkins, 2001.

Stashenko P, Yu SM. T helper and T suppressor cell reversal during the development of induced rat periapical lesion. *J. Dent. Res.* 1989; 68: 830-4.

Stashenko P. Role of immune cytokines in the pathogenesis of periapical lesions. *Endod. Dent. Traumatol.* 1990; 6: 89-96.

Summers L. The incidence of epithelium in periapical granulomas and the mechanism of cavitstion in apical dental cysts in man. *Arch. Oral. Biol.* 1974; 19: 1177-80.

Suzuki T, Kumamoto H, Kumimori K, Ooya K. Immunohistochemical analysis of apoptosis-related factors in lining epithelium of radicular cysts. *J. Oral. Pathol. Med.* 2005; 34: 46-52.

Talacko AA, Radden BG. Oral pulse granuloma: clinical and histopathological feature. A review of 62 cases. *Int. J. Oral. Maxillofacial. Surg.* 1988; 17: 343-6.

Tandri SB. Management of infected radicular cyst by surgical decompression. *J. Conserv. Dent.* 2010; 13: 159-61.

Tani-Ishii N, Kuchiba K, Osada T, et al. Effect of T-cell deficiency on the formation of periapical lesions in mice: Histological comparison between periapical lesion formation in BALB/c and BALB/c *nu/nu* mice. *J. Endod.* 1995; 21: 195-99.

Teixeira TB, Rodrigues DBR, Gervasio AM, et al. Distinct Th1, Th2 and Treg cytokines balance in chronic periapical granulomas and radicular cysts. *J. Oral. Pathol. Med.* 2010; 39: 250-6.

Teitelbaum SL. Bone resorption by osteoclasts. *Science* 2000; 289: 1504-8.

Ten Cate AR. Epithelial cell rests of Malassez and the genesis of the dental cysts. *Oral. Surg. Oral. Med. Oral. Pathol.* 1972; 34: 956-64.

Thesleff I. Epithelial cell rests of Malassez bind epidermal growth factor intensely. *J. Periodont. Res.* 1987; 33: 419-21.

Torabinejad M. The role of immunological reactions in apical cyst formation and the fate of epithelial cells after root canal therapy: a theory. *Int. J. Oral. Surg.* 1983; 12: 14-22.

Torres-Lagares D, Segura-Egea JJ, Rodriguez-Caballero A, et al. Treatment of a large maxillary cyst with marsupialization, decompression, surgical endodontic therapy and enucleation. *J. Can. Dent. Assoc.* 2011; 77: b87.

Trope M, Pettigrew J, Petras J, Barnett F, Tronstad L. Differentiation of radicular cyst and granulomas using computed tomography. *Dent. Traumatol.* 1989; 5: 69-72.

Trott JR, Chebib F, Galindo Y. Factors related to cholesterol formation in cysts and granulomas. *J. Can. Dent. Assoc.* 1973; 39: 550-5.

Valderhaug JP, Zander HA. Relationship of epithelial cell rests of Malassez to other periodontal structures. *Periodontics* 1967; 5: 254-8.

Valderhaug JP, Nylen MU. Function of epithelial rests as suggested by their ultrastructure. *J. Periodont. Res.* 1966; 1: 69-78.

Venugopal P, Kumarn A, Jyothi KN. Case series. Successful healing of periapical lesions with non-surgical endodontic approach. *J. Dent. Sci. Res.* 2011; 2: 1-6.

Wang CT, Stashenko P. Kinetics of bone resorbing activity in developing periapical lesions. *J. Dent. Res.* 1991; 70: 1362-66.

Wallström JB, Torabinejad M, Kettering J, McMilian P. Role of T cells in the pathogenesis of periapical lesions. A preliminary report. *Oral. Surg. Oral. Med. Oral. Pathol.* 1993; 76: 213-8.

Weber AL. Imaging of cysts and odontogenic tumors of the jaw. *Radiol Clin North Am.* 1993; 31: 101-20.

In: Cysts: Causes, Diagnosis and Treatment Options
Editors: A. Mendes Ortiz and A. Jimenez Moreno

ISBN: 978-1-62081-315-7
© 2012 Nova Science Publishers, Inc.

Chapter 3

CYSTIC RENAL PATHOLOGY. CLINICAL FEATURES, DIAGNOSIS AND TREATMENT OPTIONS

Francisco Javier Torres Gómez[1], Juan Manuel Poyato Galán[2], José Ramón Armas Padrón[3] and Francisco Javier Torres Olivera[1]

[1]Laboratory of Pathology and cytology Dr. Torres(CITADIAG SL), Seville, Spain
[2]Department of Urology.ClínicaSagradoCorazón, Seville, Spain
[3]Service of Pathology. Hospital UniversitarioVirgen Macarena, Seville, Spain

INTRODUCTION

The term "renal cyst" is rather non-specific because multiple entities can be subsumed within such categorization, with the same designating any cavity lined by epithelium. Will be "pseudocysts" those lesions formed by a cavity that lack of epithelial lining. In the case of a term so generic, it is difficult to calculate the actual incidence of renal cysts; however, we anticipate that this is a very frequent disease (about 5-15% of the population) [1-3].

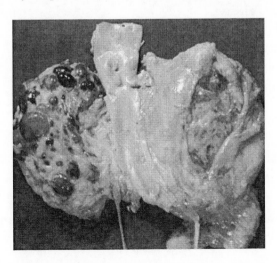

Figure 1. Multiple and bilateral cysts. Both kidneys are multilobular and reach a great size.

The pathogenesis of renal cysts may find its origin in ectatictubuli or ducts that still keep their communication with the nephron, derivating from the development of parietal diverticuli of distal or collector tubuli, or simply remain apart the glomerulus or any other nephron structure. Some theories also point out the possible action of ischemia, toxins or collagen abnormalities over the tubulus wall, as long as the effect of tubular microobstruction or tubular fluid accumulation due to glomerular filtrate and tubular fluid excretion [4-8].

Renal Cysts are a common, heterogeneous group of diseases with many clinical and radiological features and characteristics. Although their histopathology is more or less similar and constant, the number of these kidney fluid-filled pouches, their localization, their size, and their effect on the renal function will give shape to several symptomatic conditions [1-8] (Figure 1).

Historically, there have been proposed many classification systems for cysts, based on their clinical behavior, radiologic appearance or microscopic anatomy, but currently it is widely accepted the distinction between genetic and non-genetic disease1.It can be developed complicated and extensive tables qualifiers of the cystic renal pathology although the more practical approach may be made starting with the division of cysts on congenital and acquired [1-8].

Congenital cysts or dysgenesis have an unknown etiology while the influence of genetic factors is indisputable, and the performance of obstructive phenomena and tubular epithelial hyperplasia seem to have a decisive influence in its genesis.

For learning purposes we will use the following classification of cysts, compendium and variety of many other proposals from different forums:

Renal Cysts Classification

Cystic Renal Dysgenesis

- Autosomal dominant polycystic kidney disease.
- Autosomal recessive polycystic kidney disease.
- Pluricystic renal disease.
- Multicystic renal displasia.
- Medullary renal cystic disease-nephronophthisis.
- Congenitalhydronephrosis.
- Familiar hypoplasticglomerulocystic disease.

Acquired Cystic Pathology

- Acquired renal cystic disease.
- Renal simple cysts.
- Medullary sponge kidney.
- Hydronephrosis and cystic changes secondary to ureteral obstruction.
- Hemorrhagic cysts.
- Parasitic cysts.

- Sporadic glomerulocystic kidney disease.
- Calyceal diverticulum.

Neoplastic Cystic Lesions

- Cystic nephroma-multilocular cyst.
- Lymphangioma.
- Renal cell carcinoma with cystic changes.
- Other.

When it comes to addressing the study of the cystic lesions of the kidney is also important to assess the characteristics that occur in both imaging studies and in the histological study. The integration of both with clinical data will allowto define the various entities.

Cystic Renal Dysgenesis

They are a heterogeneous group of entities characterized by the presence of renal cysts related with genetic traits of inheritance, being congenital.

Autosomal Dominant Polycystic Kidney Disease

Also known as Polycystic Kidney Disease of the adult type, this is a common pathology, with an estimated incidence of 1 in every 500-1000 births. There is a genetic basis for this entity, with altered genes, PKD1(80-85%) and PKD2 (10-15%), responsible for codifying thepolycystin proteins 1 and 2, located in the chromosomes 16 and 4 (16p13.3 and 4q13-23 respectively) and a hypothetical and unknown PKD3 one (1-5%). Polycystin proteins form a calcium dependent ion chanell in the cellular membrane and are implicated in the cell cycle regulation. They are also related with renal ciliadysfunction(cilia of the distal nephron and collecting ducts) ().Prenatal diagnosis is then possible [9-12].

Cysts can be unilateral or bilateral and clinical data are not specific: flank mass (enlarged kidney) with or without pain, hematuria, hypertension (activation of the renin-angiotensin system) and renal failure (often in the end stage, 10% of the cases requiring dialysis or transplantation). Other signs and symptoms are related to infection (60%), abcess formation and lithiasis (10%). Renal cell carcinoma has been described in 2-4% of cases.

The presence of cysts in the liver in a consistent manner, and pancreatic and/or splenicones in a way occasional, confer entity of its own.There have also been described cysts in other locations such as ovaries, bladder and uterus as well as aneurysms in the basal arteries of the brain (rare). From the point of view of the image tests, simple x-ray shows imprecise kidney silhouettes. The injection of contrast allows us to observe elongation of the collecting system and "crescent" deformity of the chalices () with areas of clarity with the contrast ("Gruyère cheese").

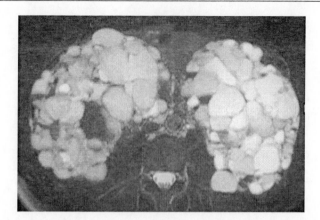

Figure 2. Autosomal Dominant Polycystic Kidney Disease; surgical piece after bilateral Nephrectomy. The patient was programmed for kidney transplantation.

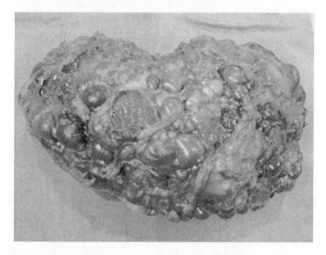

Figure 3. Coronal view of a magnetic resonance of an adult male patient with Autosomal Dominant Polycystic Kidney Disease. Bilateral renal cysts are identified in enlarged kidneys.

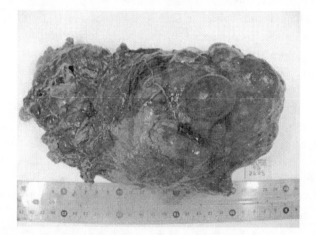

Figure 4. Autosomal dominant polycystic kidney disease (adult type). It can be appreciated nephromegaly, lobular surface and cysts of heterogeneous size, some translucent, which harbor a serous fluid, cloudy and hemorrhagic.

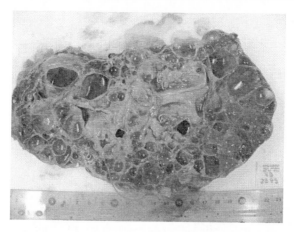

Figure 5. Autosomal dominant polycystic kidney disease (adult type). Detail of the section, with multicystic surface. No notes of renal parenchyma are seen between the cysts.

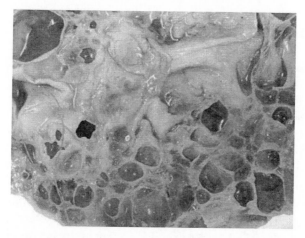

Figure 6. Autosomal dominant polycystic kidney disease (adult type). Detail of the cysts.

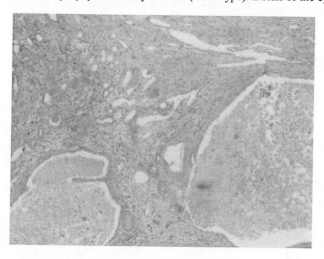

Figure 7. Autosomal dominant polycystic kidney disease (adult type). Histology. Several cysts are lined with flattened or absent epithelium. HE. 100x.

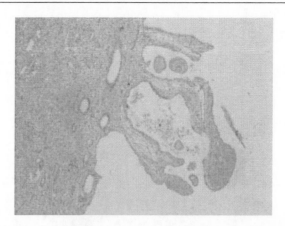

Figure8. Autosomal dominant polycystic kidney disease (adult type). Papillary projections from the cyst wall. Histology.200x.

The kidneys are increased in size due to the presence of large cystic structures that deform the renal parenchyma giving a polilobular external aspect.This macroscopic image is equivalent to that observed in the TAC, where multiple cysts with density close to that of the water is unevenly distributed (those who show an index of highest attenuation often demonstrate mucous content in the histological study) (Figures 2-6).When the disease is less severe, "normal" renal parenchyma can be seen between cysts. In severe cases, it can only be demonstrated microscopically [13-15].

Histologically, cysts of variable size are lined with flattened or cubical epithelium (Figures 7-8). Polypoid structures rising from the cyst wall can be observed. (they are not a preneoplastic condition). However, glomerular, tubular or interstitial changes are not presentuntil advanced stages in which it can be noted a common architecture with other chronic evolved nephropathies (end stage: inflammation, tubular atrophy, glomerulosclerosis, intersticial fibrosis and vascular damage). In the lumen, cysts show serous or hematicmaterial or may be observed gross calcifications that also present at the intercystic level. Lithiasis can be common (mainly urates). Stones can reach a great size, molding to the cystic wall [13-15].

Autosomal Recessive Polycystic Kidney Disease

Also known as Polycystic Kidney Disease of the infantile type, it is a rare disease (1 in every 20000 births) frequently diagnosed at early ages, being a major cause of perinatal mortality, It is associated with alterations in the gene that encodes the fibrocystin/polyductin protein, located in chromosome 6 (6p12). These alterations are also related with renal and hepatic cilia function.There is frequent association to congenital portal fibrosis. Indeed, hepatic alterations can be the main ones: hepatic cysts, portal hypertension and biliary symptoms (associated biliary dysgenesis). Renal function, usually remains preserved while those cases in which the kidneys are not functional at birth are associated with the Potter syndrome or perinatal mortality (30-50%) [9,10,16,17.

]The kidneys are increased in size leading to pulmonary hypoplasia by compression of the thoracic viscera.From the morphological point of view, the kidneys are polilobulated and spongiform(Figure 9)due to the presence of multiple medullary cysts (the most frequent, elongated) and cortical, rounded, both of them lined by flattened or cuboidal epithelium

(Figure 10). The rest of the parenchyma presents no histological alterations (Figures 11-12) until advanced stages in which the histology is shared with the chronic nephropathies [16-17].

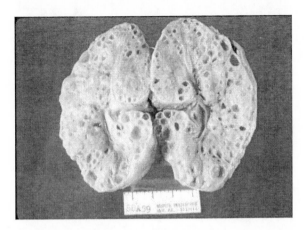

Figure 9. Autosomal reccesive polycystic kidney disease (infantile type). There is an increase of the renal size. The cut surface shows several cysts of 1-2 mm in diameter located in the cortical and medullar, acquiring the kidney a spongiform aspect.

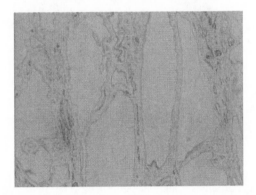

Figure 10. Autosomal reccesive polycystic kidney disease (infantile type). Histology. Cysts of different size are oriented vertically from cortex to medulla. HE.

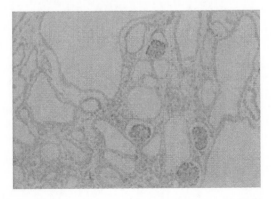

Figure 11. Autosomal reccesive polycystic kidney disease (infantile type). Histology. Normal glomeruli can be seen between cysts. HE.200x.

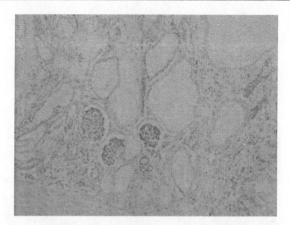

Figure 12. Autosomal reccesive polycystic kidney disease (infantile type). Histology. Cysts of different size are lined by flattened and cuboidal epithelium. Some glomeruli remain in the intercystic parenchyma. HE.200x.

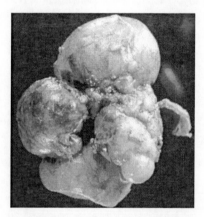

Figure 13. Multicystic renal dysplasia. There is a distortion of the renal contours, with the presence of multiple cysts that acquire a morphology "in bunch of grapes".

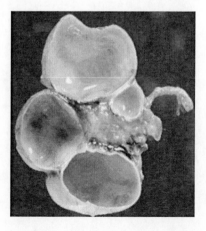

Figure 14. Multicystic renal dysplasia. Multiple and heterogeneous cysts can be seen in the renal surface. Sagital cut detail.Absence of renal parenchyma, chalices, pelvis and ureteral hypoplasia.

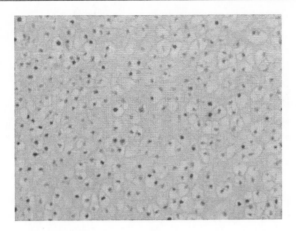

Figure 15. Multicystic renal dysplasia. Histology. Condroid elements are common. HE. 400x.

Pluricystic Renal Disease Associated with Syndromes

It is a nonspecific term used irregularly to designate the cystic changes of the kidney observed within malformation syndromes whether congenital or not. As well, kidney cysts are generally seen associated with the Down, Patau, Edward, Turner, tuberous sclerosis and Von HippelLindau syndromes.

Renal Dysplasia

The term renal dysplasia encompasses various entities that show a common characteristic such as are the alterations in the nephrogenic differentiation with an incidence of 1/4300 births). Therefore, it is not an entity by itself, but a set of alterations with different clinical manifestations and pathological features. Its presentation as cystic disease, unilateral or bilateral, allows us to bring them as renal cystic disease. In the case of embryonic disorders, it is possible to identify forms not only sporadic but also syndromic, with association with other developmental abnormalities, often of the mullerian structures. From the radiological point of view, we can identify kidney cysts that, depending on the case, will be associated or not to other abnormalities of the urinary tract. Of all the dysplasia, we are interested in those cases whose principal manifestation are renal cysts. These cysts, usually multiple,show a preferential cortical location (Figures 13-14). From the histopathological point of view these cysts are lined by a flattened or cuboidal epithelium without atypia; in the intercystic areas can be seen immature stromal tissues and heterologous elements such cartilaginous islands (Figure 15) or smooth muscle fibers (dysplastic mesenchyme) [18-22].

Medullary Cystic Kidney Disease (Cacchi-Ricchi Syndrome)

It presents characteristics superimposable to those of the nephronophthisis. In fact, it seems to be two variants of the same entity, partnering the nephronophthisis a syndromic form of autosomal recessive inheritance of renal cystic diseaseand the medullar renal cystic disease a dominant form linked to the x chromosome.

Nephronophthisis is really characterized by a heterogeneous group of mutations concerning at least six different genes (NPHP1-6) encoding nephrocystins, proteins related, like fibrocystins and polycystins, with cilia complex. On the other hand, medullary cystic kidney disease is related to MCKD1 AND MCKD2 [25-28.

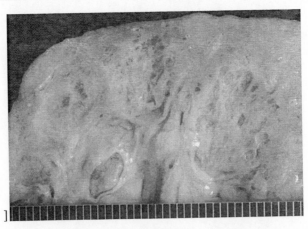

Figure16. Medullary cystic kidney disease (sponge kidney). The cysts are located at the level of medullary pyramids or are they in yuxta-medullar location, measuring from 1 to 8 mm in diameter.

While anemia, growth retardation and some symdromic manifestations (retinitis pigmentosa, hepatic and skeletal malformations, central nervous system anomalies…) are associated with nephronophthisis, hyperuricemia and gout are associated with medullary cystic kidney disease.

In any case, the morphology is similar. Both kidneys are usually affected with a reduction in size, (in medullary cystic kidney disease size can be normal)and a granular surface. The cortico-medullar junction is usually indistinct with cysts usually small in size located back to back reaching the pyramids vertex but sometimes are large enough to reach the external medullar (Figure 16).These cysts originate from the distal portions of the nephrons (loop of Henle, distal convoluted tubules and collecting ducts) and are often only identifiable microscopically. They are lined by flattened or cuboidal epithelium. Between the cysts it can be noted an axial fibrous sclerosis with glomerular and tubular atrophy (the tubules are often surrounded by a thickened basement membrane, marked in PAS stained sections) and focal or diffuse interstitial inflammation [1-8].

Congenital Hydronephrosis

While it is not a cyst by itself, it can be confused with the same on certain occasions. It is dilatation, sometimes cystic, of the renal pelvis whose more frequent causes are ureteral atresias and obstructions, mainly at the pyeloureteral junction; other etiologies and associations have been described as polar inferior artery, horseshoe kidney, extrarenal pelvis, vesicoureteralreflux, posterior ureteral valves and stenosis of the urethral meatus. It is, thus, a cavity filled with fluid that, in addition to compress the renal parenchyma of the sinus, it can be wrapped in a tissue capsule that can lead us to consider differential diagnoses, mainly in the imaging tests, with true cysts [26-28](Figure 17-18). At first, expansion of renal pelvis is protective. Then, renal failure comes.

Familiar Hypoplasticglomerulocystic Disease

Similar to acquired glomerulocystic disease, it is a rare entity characterized by glomerular cystic changes sometimes only demonstrated in microscopic studies [29-30].

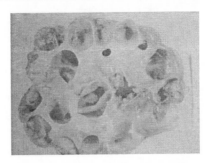

Figure 17. Massive hydronephrosis. Multiple cysts rise from renal pelvis.

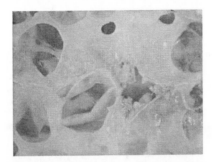

Figure 18. Massive hydronephrosis. Multiple cysts rise from renal pelvis. Detail.

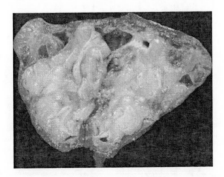

Figure 19. Acquired cystic renal disease associated with dialysis. There is an atrophic renal parenchyma with wide fatty infiltration and small cortical cysts with sizes between 0.5 and 2 cm.

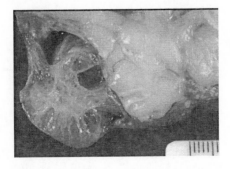

Figure 20. Acquired cystic renal disease. Detail.

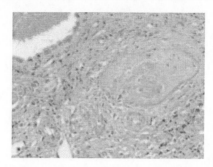

Figure 21. Final stage of renal disease. Histology. Glomerular sclerosis, tubular atrophia and inflammation. HE. 200x.

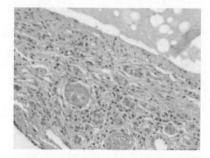

Figure 22. Final stage of renal disease. Histology. Tubular atrophia and inflammation. HE. 200x.

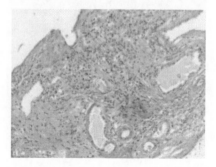

Figure 23. Final stage of renal disease. Histology. Tubular atrophia, fibrosis and architectural distortion. HE. 200x.

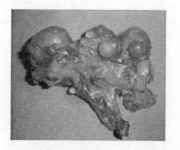

Figure 24. Small Hypodisplastic kidney with cystic disease. This young 21year-old female underwent nephrectomy due to severe recidivant Pyelonephritis.

Acquired Renal Cystic Pathology

Fibrotic disease gained more than an entity with its own personality and this is the final stage, degenerative, of different chronic nephropathies. In the case of pathologies of long evolution, the patient is usually in chronic failure and is usually subjected to dialysis, so that we should not be surprised finding references in the literature such as "nephropathy associated with dialysis". It is estimated that around 8% of patients present with some type of cyst at the time of dialysis and that virtually all the same (around 90-95 %) will have some cystic renal lesion after 10 years of dialysis. This does not mean that these lesions are symptomatic because most are subclinical being only identified in the autopsy. Cysts can be identified to cortical level and medullary (with time these are more frequent)(Figures 19-20). These are lined by cuboidal or columnar epithelium, with presence of protein or blood in the lumen. Papillary projections, sometimes with atypia can be observed raising from the cyst wall. In accordance with the terminal stage of the disease, there is widespread glomerulosclerosis, tubular atrophy and interstitial fibrosis, with a reduction in renal size [1-8, 21,22] (Figures 21-24). Acquired renal cystic pathology is related with some renal tumors, mainly papillary adenomas without clinical significance but renal cell carcinomas have also been described (6% patients in dyalisis), with papillar (the most frequent) and clear cell patterns [33].

Simple Renal Cyst (Urinary Cyst)

Radiologic studies and autopsies have shown that this is a frequent finding in kidneys of adult patients, with an estimated 50% of people older than 50 years having simple renal cysts (Figure 25), having scrounged through different etiologies such as ischaemic or infectious pathology, alterations in membrane or an origin from diverticula of the distal convoluted or collecting tubules. Its preferential location is the renal cortical,preferably at the poles less than (50-70 %) and higher (15-30 %) and may be unique (the most common situation, around 70 %) or multiple structures to cortical level, a frequent finding in imaging studies for other causes. In the simple x-ray acquire nodular morphology similar to that acquired by soft tissue lesions, with infrequent calcification. The TAC shows a well-defined mass of homogeneous density and radiolucent easily differentiable from surrounding parenchyma.

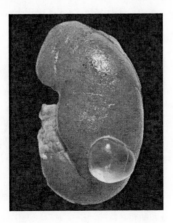

Figure 25. Simple renal cyst (urinary cyst). This is a translucent cyst with a smooth surface and serous fluid content.

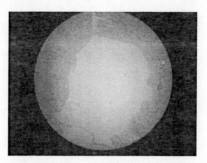

Figure 26. Simple renal cyst (urinary cyst). Histology. Central cyst and renal parenchyma without histologic alterations. HE. 40x.

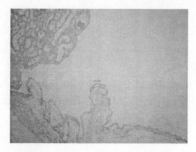

Figure 27. Simple renal cyst (urinary cyst). Histology. Cyst wall lined with cuboidal epithelium and renal parenchyma without histologic alterations. HE. 100x.

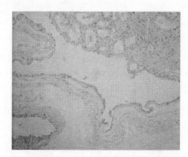

Figure 28. Simple renal cyst (urinary cyst). Histology. Cyst wall lined with cuboidal epithelium. Detail . HE. 200x.

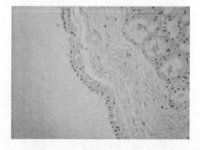

Figure 29. Simple renal cyst (urinary cyst).). Histology. Cyst wall lined with cuboidal epithelium. Detail . HE. 200x.

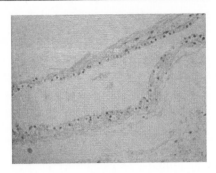

Figure 30. Simple renal cyst (urinary cyst).). Histology. Cyst wall lined with cuboidal epithelium. Detail . HE. 200x.

Radiological criteria that define the simple renal cyst have shown great sensitivity and diagnostic specificity provided that they will be followed with severity [7]:

- Mass without echogenicity in its interior walls.
- smooth and well-defined posterior acoustic shadowing.
- Shadows along the edges of the reinforcement later.

Histologically they are simple isolated cysts lined by flattened or cuboidal epithelium without alteration of the parenchymal intercystic structures (Figures 26-30). This is an asymptomatic finding in most occasions although cases have been described with complications such as hemorrhage, infection, the increase in size and even the development of neoplastic foci (concomitant finding) [34-36].

Medullary Sponge Kidney

Tubular ectasia of the collecting ducts originates cystic structures at the level of medullary pyramids giving a spongiform aspect to the kidney depending of the severity of the changes. If the cysts reach a great size, renal contours can be disturbed (pronounced spongiform changes). On the other hand, cysts can only be seen microscopically. They are multiple, small and limited to pyramids and papillae in a diffuse or focal manner. The epithelium is flattened or cuboidal but it can be columnar.Cyst are usually connected with collecting tubules. The intercystic parenchyma is frequently altered, with presence of inflammation, tubular atrophy and scarring [37,38,39,40].

Symptoms are related to lithiasis, infection or hematuria.

Hydronephrosis and Ectatic Changes Secondary to Obstruction of the Urinary Tract

While it is not a matter of cystic pathology by itself, its morphology can remember cystic structures with which it will be necessary to establish a differential diagnosis. Obstruction of the urinary tract is often not complete but ectatic changes that occur proximally to obstruction can acquire cystic morphology. This is the case with hydronephrosis and pyelectasis and calyceal (Figure 31). Mere dilations, the urinary tract retains its lining urothelialsurface while the epithelium can display various degrees of thinning. From the radiologicaland macroscopic point of view, renal architecture is generally respected; the lesion is located in renal pelvis or calyceallevel [1-8, 41].

Hemorrhagic Cyst

It is a collection of blood inintracapsularor intraparenchymallocation, usually cortical. While it is a rare finding whose main etiology is a trauma, in 25% of the cases is associated to tumor. Sonographically there are echoes and internal lack of reinforcement later while it is sometimes difficult to make a distinction with regard to neoplastic lesions. Histologically they are constituted by bloodymaterial [42-43](Figure 32).

Parasitic Cysts

Its incidence is estimated at around 2 %, usually secondary to hematogenous extension of an infestation from another location. The simple radiology can demonstrate calcification override intraparenchymatous while the TAC will show, in general, a cystic thick wall enhanced by the contrast. The ultrasound study, on the other side, will prove a cystic lesion with mixed echogenicity.

Hydatid cyst, the most common, is caused by the larval or cystic stage of echinococcus tapeworms, being echinococcusgranulosusthe most common. Histologically, the cyst wall can be surrounded by a fibrous capsule, sometimes calcified, or granulation tissue and is composed by an inner germinal layer and an external fibrous and laminar layer. The cyst is filled with serous-like fluid containing, when viable (no calcification), daughter cysts and brood capsules with scolices [44-45].

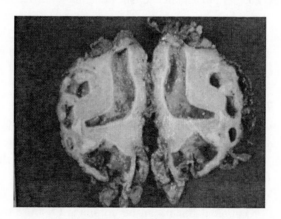

Figure 31. Hydronephrosis secondary to ureteral obstruction.

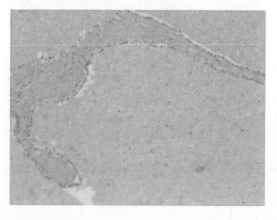

Figure 32. Hematic cyst. Hystology. HE.200x.

Sporadic (Acquired) Glomerulocystic Kidney Disease

It is a rare entity in which cortical cyst are the result of dilatation of the Bowman's capsula and glomerular atrophy, probably secondary to ischemic lesions leading to proximal tubular obstruction. Only a hand of cases have been described, most of them associated with different systemic diseases (hemolytic-uremic syndrome, prolonged peritoneal dialysis, severe hypertension…)

Some lesions are only demonstrated histologically. Bowman's spaces are dilated and glomerular vases are atrophic [46-50].

Calyceal Diverticulum

It is a cystic eventration of the upper urinary tract lying in the renal parenchyma communicating with the collectinc system through a narrow channel. It is an uncommon entity with an incidence of 2-4 cases per 1000 intravenous urogram examinations. While calyceal diverticula are rare, stone formation within them is frequent. Histologically, calyceal cyst is lined by cuboidal or flattened epithelium depending the grade of dilation [50-54].

Renal Neoplasms with Cystic Changes

Virtually all kidney tumors can display cystic changes. However, there are entities being the most obvious and frequent. On them we will emphasize in this section [55-57].

Cystic Nephroma (Multilocular Cyst)

Many are the authors who grouped the cystic nephromaalong with cystic nephroblastoma, arguing that these are two manifestations of the same entity, differentiated in essence to histological level by the presence or absence of blastemal. Although the cystic nephroblastomais associated with early ages, the cystic nephromahas been described in both children and adults. It is a benign cystic neoplasm, well demarcated from the adjacent parenchyma (encapsulated), composed of cystic cavities of heterogeneous size (from millimeters to few centimeters) lined by flattened or cuboidal epithelium. The intercystic septa can be fibrous, although sometimes in them It can be seen kidney structures without histologicalterations; it is also common notto find them, still the fibrous septa adapted to the cystic cavities. The correct identification of these elements will be of crucial importance for differentialdiagnosis with cystic carcinomas in which neoplastic elements can be identified in this location. The absence of parenchymatous elements will allow in most of the occasions solve the problems of differential diagnosis with congenital polycystic kidney diseases being possible to observe parenchymatous elements without histologic alterations.58-59 The cystic nephroma is a benign tumor whose treatment of choice is surgical excision and whose prognosis is excellent. Those cases in which has been described recurrence have been incompletely excised.

Lymphangioma

It is a benign tumor of lymphatic origin consisting of a cystic dilatation lined by endothelium, hyperplastic or not hyperplastic, in whose lumen is usually observed a serous fluid (usually corresponding to lymph, without the presence of erythrocytes). This can be a single lesion or they can be multiple, located mostly at the level of the renal sinus (polycystic disease of the renal sinus) being the cortical locations (second in frequency) and medullary(less frequent) but equal to or more conflict in what the differential diagnosis is concerned, especially when the injury reaches large size. The presence of multiple lesions, usually of small size, willing diffusely in the renal parenchyma, receives the name of lymphangiomatosis. There are cases associated with dilatations of lymph vessels in the perirenal tissues generally associated with ascites [60-62].

Multilocular Cystic Renal Cell Carcinoma

Its name is extremely descriptive. This is a variant of clear cell renal cell carcinoma that acquires personality of its own, and therefore has been registered as an independent entity in the WHO classification of 200455. The neoplasm, generally well delimited of the adjacent renal parenchyma (there is usually a capsule or inflammatorycells) is made up of multiple cysts of heterogeneous size that harbor a serous fluid or blood. The cysts are separated by septa in which can be identified clear carcinoma cells of low grade atypia. These are, at times, scarce and difficult to identify which is why it is always advisable to make serial sections in order to identify neoplastic cells, being able to perform a correct classification (with prognostic value). Because the clear cell renal cell carcinoma may show cystic changes, the differential diagnosis between the two entities will be based principally on the extension of the cystic change, and the architecture and cytology of cells; if the changes are extensive, it will be a multilocular cystic carcinoma; in that case we will observe the architecture of the neoplasm: if atypia is of low grade and the cells are available in rows, surely we are faced with amultilocular cystic carcinoma. If there is high-gradeatypia and/or neoplastic cells are arranged in expansive nests, the diagnosis of clear cell carcinoma is favored. Sometimes we can consider the differential diagnosis between clear cell carcinoma and histiocytes with clear cytoplasm, especially in those cases in which the tumor cells are scarce and its disposal is isolated. The immunohistochemistry is a weapon of great diagnostic value because the cells of the renal cell carcinoma are positive for EMA and cytokeratins and negative for CD68, positive marker in histiocytes. Surgery is still sufficient: simple nephrectomy. The prognosis is usually excellent in spite of having been described recurrences or metastases [1-8,63,64].

Cystic Nephroblastoma

It also deserves its inclusion as an independent entity in the WHO classification of 2004. The term defines it as partially differentiated cysticnephroblastoma. It is a neoplasm of childhood (the majority of patients have an age under two yearsalthough it can also be manifested in the adult).As in the case of multilocular cystic renal cell carcinoma, this tumor is composed of the apposition of cysts lined by cuboidal, flat or hobnail cells, and may even be absent such lining. The characteristic feature lies in the identification of own structures of nephroblastoma in intercystic septa, i.e. blastemal, stroma (usually immature) and epithelial elements (also immature, tubular or papillary-glomerular). In the case of a morphological variant of the nephroblastoma (Wilms' Tumor), the diagnostic features, therapeutic and prognosis are the same [1-8,65-67].

Papillary Renal Cell Carcinoma

At times, the cystic cavities located between the papillary structures can reach a great size, giving rise to a mixed neoplasm, cystic and papillary. However, those changes are considered a macroscopic variant not deserving to be classified as an independent entity. Of course, their therapeutic characteristics and prognosisdoes not differ from those exhibited by the common papillary carcinoma. Exceptional entities that can cause problems in diagnosis with renal neoplasms with cystic changes have been described in the literature, usually as isolated cases. We emphasize the report of an intraparenchymatoUSneurysm of the renal artery whose wall had a re-channelledthrombus that was interpreted as tumor in the imaging tests7. After the nephrectomy, the surgical specimen showed the true nature of the lesion [1-8].

Others

Other benign tumors may likewise to exhibit cystic changes with sufficient relevance as to raise differential diagnoses with cystic carcinomas. As well, we wish to highlight cases of urinary adenomas with cystic predominance, cystic angiomyolipomas [68], metanephric adenomas [69] and cystic oncocytomas [70]. A renal artery aneurysm has been described mimicking cystic renal cell carcinoma [71].The cystic changes are relatively common in the kidney, joining or not to neoplasms and/or tumors. Their structural or degenerative nature allows us to observe them in countless situations so the list of these would be endless. In summary, before the identification of renal cystic structures it will be necessary to observe the histological characteristics of the lining epithelium in order to look for histologic features that identify a neoplasia. It will then have to discard such features at the level of the interseptalstroma. Treatment and prognosis derived from the identification of the same will be of the greatest clinical significance.

ADDENDUM: DIAGNOSIS AND TREATMENT OPTIONS OF RENAL CYSTS

Diagnosis

Nowadays, and due to the high resolution standards of the antenatal detection techniques, the very first diagnostic approach to the cystic disease should be based on in utero findings. The simple presence of fetal oligohydramnios in pregnant regular ultrasound examinations simultaneously with enlarged homogeneously hypoechogenic kidneys, might be strongly in association with such disorder.

As generally cysts are asymptomatic, in adults they are incidentally discovered when a sonography or a scan is performed due to an abdominal or pelvic problem.

In this second case, under ultrasound observation cysts appear as round or oval-shaped sacs, with a smooth surface sharply defined by a thin wall which contains internal anechoic fluid with no visible tracts and a posterior acoustic enhancement. Presence of internal echoes, bad transmission of ultrasound waves or irregular perimeter would lead to perform further evaluation (CT or even sharp needle aspiration) to discharge complications or malignancies. These special conditions are summarized under the well knownBosniak classification of simple and complex cysts (Figures 33-39) [72,73].

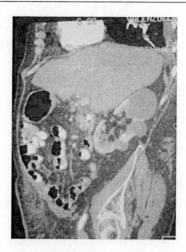

Figure 33. Renal sonogram of a simple benign cyst. Bosniak I.

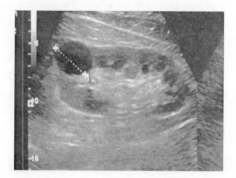

Figure 34. Front view of a magnetic resonance showing bilateral simple cysts. Bosniak I.

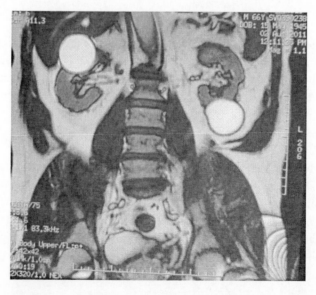

Figure 35. Renal sonogram of an uncomplicated renal cyst with minimal septation and calcification. Bosniak II.

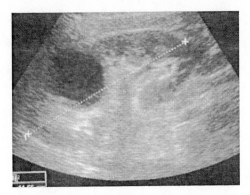

Figure 36. Computed tomographic scan of a hyperdense cyst of the upper pole of a left kidney. Bosniak IIF.

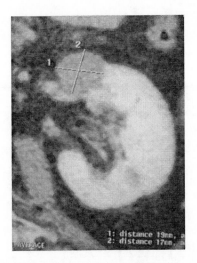

Figure 37. Renal sonogram of a complex cyst, with strong calcifications, more prominent septations, a thicker wall than a category II lesion and even an intracystic fluid level suggesting bleeding or infection; more likely to be benign than malignant but highly suspicious.Requires surgical exploration and/or removal.

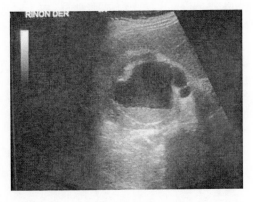

Figure 38. Lateral view of a magnetic resonance showing multiple uncomplicated benign cysts in a sane kidney.

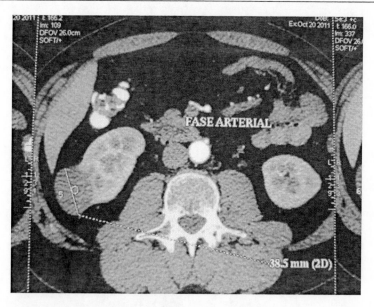

Figure 39. Computed tomographic scan of a Bosniak IV renal cyst.

Category I	Simple benigncystwith:
	Good through transmission (i.e. acoustic enhancement).
	No echoes within the cyst.
	Sharply, marginated smooth wall.
	Requires NO surgery.
Category II	Looks benign with some radiologic concerns including septation, minimal
	calcification, and high density
Category IIF	Minimal Atypia. Requires NO surgery.
	More than three septations, strong calcification. Hyperdense Cyst.
	SignificativeAtypia. Requires NO surgery.
Category III	More complicated lesion that cannot confidently be distinguished from
	malignancy, having more calcification, more prominent septation of a thicker
	wall than a category II lesion; more likely to be benign than malignant.
	Suspicious Cyst. Requires surgical exploration and/or removal.
Category IV	Clearly a malignant lesion with large cystic components, irregular margins,
	solid vascular elements.
	Very Suspicious Cyst. Requires surgical removal.

CT scan criteria are quite similar to those applied to sonography except for including density ranges considered physiological (between -10 and +20 Hounsfield Units). Hyperdense values between 20 and 90HU should suggest a simple cyst if no enhancement is observed during the intravenous injection of contrast fluid, while positive response in the way of a strong enhancement would translate the presence of blood vessels and therefore the possibility of a neoplasm.

Complicated cysts are those containing calcifications, fluids, pus or blood, and in the same case of border-line lesions, require more studies such as needle puncture/biopsy or MRI to discharge a Cystic Neoplasm. The puncture should give some histological data, but the MRI does not offer much information in comparison with the CT if not for its specificity identifying the nature of the fluids, which is important because between 5-10% of Renal Neoplasms can present a liquid content mass appearance [73,74].

Needle biopsy performance is sometimes controversial when indicated prior to surgery exploration. Although it is considered a relatively safe diagnostic procedure complications can occur, particularly in less experienced hands. Furthermore, the procedure is unnecessary in many of the patients in which it is performed. Certainly, in the case of suspicious renal cysts renal biopsy should not be used because the imaging study (that was performed for diagnosis) is inadequate. Also, besides the complications of bleeding, infection, or needle track tumor spread, a negative biopsy result does not rule out malignancy; particularly in cystic lesions have less bulk of tissue to sample.Anyway, in the words of other authors, although some individuals do not biopsy cystic renal lesions because of the potential for false-negative results and risk for tumor seeding, at some recognized institutions all Bosniak type III lesions undergo biopsy before surgery because up to 39% of lesions categorized as category III can be benign [75,76,77].

Currently there are no randomized controlled trials with regarding to follow-up or management of cystic renal masses, as such, the recommendations are primarily expert opinion78. At this time, category I and II renal cysts do not require further imaging or follow-up. Patients in category IIF, because of the approximate 5% malignant risk, do require periodic imaging (there is no consensus or evidence based interval determined for follow-up imaging). And combination of ultrasound and MRI should be considered as follow-up for Bosniak IIF and reduces the lifetime radiation dose (once that the lesion has been characterized by triphasic CT scan) in patients younger than 50 years. For category III (50% malignant risk) and category IV (75% to 90% malignant risk) surgical excision is recommended (Evidence Level 3, Recommendation Grade B). Although MRI may add further information, it should be used as an adjunct to CT scans in difficult cases (Level 4 evidence, Grade C recommendation) [79,80].

Apart from the risk of being a step of the expression of a malignancy, when the cysts are multiple, diffuse or bilateral, the option of an Autosomal Dominant Polycystic Kidney Disease must be kept in mind, and family/genetic studies should be performed too.

Anyway, every extremely complicated cyst or strongly suspicious lesion must undergo surgical exploration avoiding the subjectivity of the imaging.

Surgical Treatment Options

The clinical features of the cystic uncomplicated diseases remain generally asymptomatic for they do not produce any manifestation, which means that no therapeutic attitude should be adopted. In cases of large cysts the compression effect could cause pyelocalyceal obstructions or even hypertension, but the most common signs are abdominal pain, flank mass palpation or even hematuria (secondary to a penetration of the cyst in the renal pelvis).

In the case of percutaneous drainage of solitary kidney cysts followed by injection of pure alcohol, as a sclerotic agent, there are some evidenced studies that state this option as an effective therapeutic method with only a few complications; however it is not always effective and can pose a risk of fibrosis when perihilar cysts are approched [81,82].

The definitive treatment of the complex cystic disease is always surgical and the reference techniques are the puncture-aspiration followed by sclerotherapy, the laparoscopic unroofing or removal of the cyst, either transperitoneally or retroperitoneally, and the partial/radical laparoscopic nephrectomy in cases of a highly suspected neoplastic component of the cyst.

The laparoscopic approach in comparison with conventional open surgery means an important step in the development of minimally invasive techniques. Recent laparoscopic kidney surgery series have shown that patients benefit from shorter hospital stays, less pain, and an earlier return to normal activities. Furthermore, some reported advantages of retroperitoneal access include quicker access to the renal hilum, easier dissection in obese individuals, the avoidance of intraperitoneal irritation, and less interference with ventilatory and hemodynamic function [83].

For the transperitoneal laparoscopic approach the procedure steps include:

- Trocar placement and renal exposure as conventionally.
- Careful management and movilization of duodenum in case of right-sided dissections.
- Opening of Gerota´s fascia to better expose the cyst.
- Needle aspiration of the cyst (the aspired liquid is sent to cytopathologic study).
- Excision of the cyst wall (also sent to pathologic analysis).
- Biopsy of the cyst base and parenchymal surface (also sent to pathologic interpretation).
- Completion of cyst decortication.
- Performance of partial/radical nephrectomy in case that malignancies are found in the specimens sent to pathologic consideration.

For the retroperitoneal laparoscopic approach the procedure steps vary:

- Trocar placement in the posterior axillary line.
- Establishment of a pneumoretroperitoneum.
- Identification of anterior wall after dissection of retroperitoneal fat.
- Exposition of the kidney lower pole and posterior surface by up-tractioning the perinephric fat (Kocher maneuver).
- Rest of procedure as described for transperitoneal access [84].

Today, laparoscopic surgery is being increasingly used for a large variety of ablative and reconstructive procedures of the urinary tract, including the management of cysts, and brand new instruments/procedures emerge almost weekly. Standard laparoscopy has evolutioned both to hand-assisted proceedings (using the surgeon´s hand for retraction and dissection) and single-port techniques (only one skin incision instead of three to six ports). These two innovations reduce access-related morbidity and improve the cosmetic outcome of laparoscopic surgery avoiding the use of several and larger (5 mm, 10-12 mm) ports inserted through big sized skin incisions, and the necessary triangulation of the surgeon's right- and left-hand instruments for the surgical dissection (Figures 40-41) [85].

But efforts are continuing to reach further. These include the use of mini-laparoscopic 2 mm needle-ports, also known as needlescopicports, that have almost no cosmetic sequelae and do not increase the morbidity of the surgical procedure. These fine instruments can be passed through 2 mm Veress needle-ports that are about the diameter of a 16G angiocath needle, are designed to be inserted with no need for a skin incision, which means they do not require formal closure, and are associated with negligible scarring or pain [85].

In the same way, the use of natural orifices (Natural Orifice Transluminal Endoscopic Surgery= NOTES) has recently generated intense interest in the scientific community, in order to perform nephrectomy and other kidney surgery completely avoiding abdominal wall incisions and attendant scarring. Transvaginal access is the worldwide most frequently used NOTES approach to date, but although the technique may be safely performed for the abdominal wall remains intact, the potential for complications should not be ignored. The close proximity of structures like rectum, ureters or even small intestine (with its tendency to occupy the pelvis) should be considered while thinking about this therapeutic feasible option. Rectum-colonic injuries, small bowel lacerations, ureterovaginal fistula formation, vulvar damage and bladder injuries have been reported for NOTES proceeding, confirming that independently of the minimally invasive access intra-abdominal, damage is expected to be the same as it depends on mobilization of the target organ, its adjacent viscera and parieties [86,87,88].

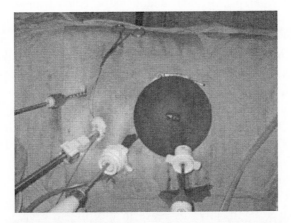

Figure 40. Spatial disposition of the laparoscopic ports ready for a hand-assisted kidney surgery.

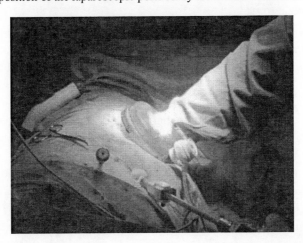

Figure 41. Introduction of the hand through the transperitoneal access while using the camera to help in the dissection of the kidney.

Anyway, in the concrete case of renal cysts at the moment there are not enough evidences in terms of a large number of treated cases to analyze, corresponding the majority of the reported studies to renal tumours. In years to come, as long as technological progress develop less aggressive and cheaper tools, NOTES will surely be an option to keep in mind not only for reference institutions but for every hospital with experience in laparoscopic performance.

Non Surgical Treatments Options

No cure has been still found for genetic diseases like Autosomal Recessive Polycystic Kidney Disease (ARPKD or Infantile Form), so the main aim of the treatment should focus on the management of the complications inherent to this disease. In case of surviving patients (30% of affected infants die immediately in the neonatal period or during the first year of life principally due to respiratory insufficiency and/or lung infections) it is known they will progress to a severe renal failure (End Stage Renal Disease= ESRD) along the first decade of life in an approximately 50% of the cases, so early neonatal respiratory care and kidney function replacement therapies would undoubtedly help increasing the possibility of improving their long-term survival rates. Concomitant therapies to manage hypertension, congestive heart failure, hepatosplenomegaly and portal hypertension should also be performed [89,90]. Considering these aspects, the ten-year survival of those who live beyond the first year of life has improved to 82%, fifteen-year survival is estimated to be 67%-79%, and may be improving [91].

When talking about the Autosomal Dominant Polycystic Kidney Disease (ADPKD or Adult Form), one of the most common monogenic disorders and globally the third most common cause of ESRD, there must be said that studies carried out during the last decade have suggested new horizons in the possibility of slowing cyst growth [92,93,94]. Although there is no specific treatment the measures begin with the standard support therapies for chronic renal disease, as control of Hypertension and Dyslipidaemia, with very promising studies that point out a significative decrease in the protein excretion when Angiotensin Converting Enzime inhibitors (ACEi) are used [95,96]but a faster loss of renal function when Diuretics were received [97].

On the other hand, the use of Statins has shown to be a good tool in the fight against the progression of the disease while Dyslipidaemia is a risk progression factor. These HMG-CoA reductase inhibitors have several functions (inhibition of proliferation of a number of kidney cell lines, induction of apoptosis, inhibition of chymokine and cytokine release by mesangial cells and monocytes, and inhibition of matrix components by mesangial cells) [98,99] and its use has suggested an action on the endothelial function of the kidney regarding a better renal plasma flow and a significative vasodilator response to Acetylcholine in the forearm [100].

As it is known that patients with ADPKD suffer an overexpression of c-myc oncogene, associated with apoptosis and probed to induce renal cyst in transgenic mice, Antisense oligonucleotides should be used to inhibit expression of overexpressed mRNAs to inhibit the progression of the disease [101-106].

Among other changes consistently found in ADPKD cells is activation of the Ser/Thr kinase mammalian target of rapamycin (mTOR), an enzyme that coordinates cell growth, cell-cycle progression, and proliferation [38], and Sirolimus (originally referred to as Rapamycin) is a macrocyclic lactone that is derived from Streptomyces Hygroscopicus and exerts antiproliferative and growth-inhibiting effects as well as antifibrotic effect by inhibition of the mTOR enzyme [107-108]. When used in comparison with conventional treatments, Sirolimus halted cysts growth and increased parenchimal volume suggesting a good effect that must be followed up in the future supported by forthcoming research [109].

Somatostatin has been recently studied too as a prevention of ADPKD progression based on a clinical observation, significantly slowing kidney volume increase, but longer and larger clinical trials will be necessary to establish the long-term safety and efficacy of somatostatin analogs for ADPKD and/or ADPLD [110-111].

Although many clinical trials are underway and preliminary results are not yet available, there is an increasingly interest on the effect of the Vasopressin Antagonists over the ADPKD, and the target of the in-course research is to.

Alterations in intracellular calcium homeostasis and cAMP (cyclic adenosine 3',5'-phosphate) support the increased cell proliferation and fluid secretion in cystic epithelia, but there are several hormone receptors acting as cellular mediators which can stimulate cAMP increase [112-113]. These receptors that are preferentially expressed in affected tissues are the logical treatment targets, and as some animal studies demonstrated abnormalities of Vasopressin and Vasopressin receptors, which could result in increased intracellular cAMP generation, research was performed (with Vasopressin V2-receptor antagonists OPC-31260 and Tolvaptan, initially developed for other clinical purposes) to inhibit the development of ADPKD in different animal models. In vivo studies observed a slow curse in animals with ADPKD but human clinical trials in patients with ADPKD treated with Tolvaptan, are under way trying to demonstrate that cAMP can promote ADPKD progression [114-115].

As a final point, in the therapeutic management of other acquired cystic renal diseases the general recommendations are:

- Acquired Renal Cystic Disease (ARCD): Light Hematuria episodes should be expected, and can be handled with bed rest, antimicrobial and analgesics.
- Medullary Sponge Kidney (MSK): The most important attitude is to recommend patients to increase the liquids intake over 2 liters per day, especially in those suffering from Nephrolithiasis, and promote Urinary Infections preventive measures. Oral Thiazidediureticswillbenefitpatientswith active Hypercalciuria.
- Simple Cyst: The infection of one of these cysts should be managed with a combination of antimicrobial and, when complicated, surgical approach.

REFERENCES

[1]   Zhou M., Magi-Galluzzi C., editors. *Genitourinary Pathology, a volume in the series Foundations in Diagnostic Pathology*. Elsevier. Churchill Livingstone 2007. US.

[2]   Algaba F., Moreno A., Trias I. *Uropatología no tumoral. Correlación morfológica, molecular y clínica. Firstedition.* Pulso editions. 1997. Barcelona.

[3]   Murphy WM., Beckwith JB., Farrow GM., editors of Tumors of the Kidney, Bladder and Related Urinary Structures. *Atlas of Tumor Pathology*. Third series. AFIP.1994. Washington.

[4]   Berstein J., Gilbert-Barness E. *Developmental Abnormalities of the Kidney, in Diagnostic Surgical Pathology,* edited by Sternberg S. Second edition. Raven Press 1994. New York.

[5]   Peces R., Costero O. El espectro de los quistes renales en el adulto: diagnóstico diferencial y complicaciones. *Nefrología* 2003(3): 260-65.

[6]   Bisceglia M., Galliani CA., Senger C., Stallone C., Sessa A. Renal cystic diseases: a review. *Adv. Anat. Pathol.* 2006; 13(1): 26-56.

[7]   Levine E., Hartman DS., Meilstrup JW., Van Slyke MA., Edgar KA., Barth JC. Current concepts and controversies in imaging of renal cystic diseases. *Urol. Clin. North Am.* 1997; 24(3):523-43.

[8]   Thomsen HS., Levine E., Meilstrup JW., Van Slyke MA., Edgar KA., Barth JC et al. Renal Cystic diseases. *Eur. Radiol.* 1997; 7(8): 1267-75.

[9]   Waters AM., Beales PL. Ciliopathies: an expanding disease spectrum.*Pediatr_Nephrol.* 2011 Jul; 26(7):1039-56. Epub 2011 Jan 6.

[10]   Gunay-Aygun M. Liver and kidney disease in ciliopathies.*Am. J. Med. Genet. C. Semin. Med. Genet.* 2009 Nov 15; 151(4):296-306.

[11]   Karihaloo A., Koraishy F., Huen SC, Lee Y., Merrick D., Caplan MJ., Somlo S., Cantley LG. Macrophages promote cyst growth in polycystic kidney disease.*J. Am. SocNephrol.* 2011 Oct; 22(10):1809-14. Epub 2011 Sep 15.

[12]   Bergmann C., Von Bothmer J., Ortiz Bruchle N., Venghaus A., Frank V., Fehrenbach H. et al.Mutations in multiple PKD genes may explain early and severe polycystic kidney disease. *J. Am. Soc. Nephrol.* 2011; 22(11): 2047-56.

[13]   Al-Bhalal L., Akhtar M. Molecular basis of autosomal dominant polycystic kidney disease. *Adv. Anat. Pathol.* 2005; 12(3):126-33.

[14]   Harris PC. Autosomal dominant polycystic kidney disease: clues to pathogenesis. *Hum. Mol. Genet.* 1999; 8(10):1861-6.

[15]   Veldhuisen B., Spruit L., Dauwerse HG., Breuning MH., Peters DJ. Genes homologous to the autosomal dominant polycystic kidney disease genes (PKD1 and PKD2). *Eur. J. Hum. Genet.* 1999 Dec; 7(8):860-72.

[16]   Sweeney WE., Avner ED. Molecular and cellular pathophysiology of autosomal recessive polycystic kidney disease (ARPKD). *Cell. Tissue. Res.* 2006; 326(3): 671-85.

[17]   Al-Bhalal L., Akhtar M. Molecular basis of autosomal recessive polycystic kidney disease (ARPKD). *Adv. Anat. Pathol.* 2008; 15(1): 54-58.

[18]   Schreuder MF., Westland R., van Wijk JA. Unilateral multicystic dysplastic kidney: a meta-analysis of observational studies on the incidence, associated urinary tract malformations and the contralateral kidney. *Nephrol. Dial Transplant.* 2009; 24(6): 1810-18.

[19]   Kuwertz-Broeking E., Brinkmann OA., von Lengerke HJ., Sciuk J., Fruend S., Bulla M. et al. Unilateral multicystic dysplastic kidney: experience in children. *BJU* 2004; 93(3): 388-92.

[20]   Psooy K. Multicystic dysplastic kidney in the neonate: the role of the urologist. *Can. Urol. Assoc. J.* 2010; 4(2): 95-97.

[21] Arena S., Fazzari C., Scuderi MG., Implantini A., Villari D., Torre S., Arena F. et al. Molecular events included in the morphogenesis of multicystic dysplastic kidney. *Urol. Int.* 2010; 85(1): 106-11.

[22] Harambat J., Dobremez E., Llanas B. What is new in dysplastic multicystic kidney disease?. *Arch. Pediatr.* 2009; 16(6): 696-97.

[23] Hurd TW., Hildebrandt F. Mechanisms of nephronophthisis and related ciliopathies. *Nephron. Exp. Nephrol.* 2011; 118(1): 9-14.

[24] Hildebrandt F., Attanasio M., Otto E. Nephronophthisis: disease mechanisms of a ciliopathy. *J. Am. Soc. Nephrol.* 2009; 20(1): 23-35.

[25] Wolf MT., Hildebrandt F. Nephronophthisis. *Pediatr. Nephrol.* 2011; 26(2): 181-94.

[26] Bosoteanu M., Bosoteanu C., Deacu M., Aschie M., Bordei P. Etio-pathogenic and morphological correlations in congenital hydronephrosis. *Rom. J. Morphol. Embryol.* 2011; 52(1): 129-36.

[27] Delgado-Plasencia L., Hernández-Siverio N., Castro Díaz D. Prenatal hydronephrosisduetocongenitalureteralvalves. *Actas Urol. Esp* 2010; 34(7): 643-45.

[28] Bekele W., Sánchez TR. Congenital megacalyces presenting as neonatal hydronephrosis. *Pediatr. Radiol* 2010; 40(9): 1579.

[29] Sharp CK., Bergman SM., Stockwin JM., Robbin ML., Galliani C., Guay-Woodford LM. Dominantly transmitted glomerulocystic kidney disease. A distinct genetic entity. *J. Am. Soc. Nephrol.* 1997; 8(1): 77-84.

[30] Dedeoglu IO., Fisher JE., Springate JE., Waz WR., Stapleton FB., Feld LG. Spectrum of glomerulocystic kidneys: a case report and review of the literature. *Pediatr. Pathol. Lab. Med.* 1996; 16(6): 941-49.

[31] Levine E. Acquired cystic kidney disease. *Radiol. Clin. North Am*. 1996; 34: 947-64.

[32] Mickisch O., Bommer J., Bachmann S., Waldherr R., Mann JFE., Ritz E. Multicystic transformation of kidneys in chronic renal failure. *Nephron.* 1984; 38: 93-99.

[33] Fleming S. Renal cell carcinoma in acquired cystic kidney disease. *Histopathology* 2010, 56(5): 395-400.

[34] Murshidi MM., Suwan ZA. Simple renal cysts. *Arch. Esp. Urol*. 1997; 50: 928-31.

[35] Terada N., Ichioka K., Matsuda Y., Okubo K., Yoshimura K., Arai Y. The natural history of simple renal cysts. *J. Urol.* 2002; 167: 21-23.

[36] Baert L., Steg A. Is the diverticulum of the distal and collecting tubules a preliminary stage of the simple cyst in the adult?. *J. Urol.* 1977; 118: 707-10.

[37] Pritchard MJ. Medullary sponge kidney: causes and treatments. *Br. J. Nurs.* 2010; 19(15): 972-76.

[38] Stratta P., Fenoglio R., Quaglia M., Lazzarich E., Airoldi A. The missing medullary sponge kidney. *Kidney Int.* 2009; 76(4): 459-60.

[39] Stratta P., Canavese C., Lazzarich E., Fenoglio R., Morellini V., Quaglia M. et al. Medullaryspongekidney. *Am. J. Kidney Dis.* 2006; 48(6): 87-88.

[40] Lee S., Jang YB., Kang KP., Kim W., Park SK. Medullary sponge kidney. *Kidney int.* 2006; 70(6): 979.

[41] Shiao CC., Tsai CC., Huang CH., Yang CL., Kao JL. Duplex kidney with giant hydronephrosis presenting as huge cysts. *Nephrology* 2011; 16(4): 453.

[42]   Pérez Fontán FJ., Pombo Felipe F., Ruiz Fontán J., Comesaña ML. Hemorrhagic cyst mimicking renal malignancy in a child. *Ann. Radiol.* 1993; 36(2): 142-44.

[43]   Quiñones Ortiz L., Guerediaga Madariaga J., Fernández SimónJM., Guate Ortiz JL., Escaf Barmadah S. Castellanos González L. et al. Acquired cystic renal disease. A case report of intracystichemorrahage simulating renal tumor. *Arch. Esp. Urol.* 1994; 47(1): 76-78.

[44]   Ballesteros Sampol JJ. Renal hydatidiccyst. *Actas. Urol. Esp.* 2006; 30(9): 967.

[45]   Abascal Junquera JM., Esquena Fernández S., Martos Calvo R., Ramírez Sevilla C., Salvador Lacambra C., Celma Doménech A. et al. Renal hydatidiccystsimulatinghypernephroma. *Actas. Urol. Esp.* 2005; 29(2): 233-25.

[46]   Emma F., Muda AO., Rinaldi S., Boldrini R., Bosman C., Rizzoni G. Acquired glomerulocystic kidney disease following hemolytic-uremic syndrome. *Pediat. Nephrol.* 2001; 16(7): 557-60.

[47]   Vera-Sempere F., Zamora I., Simon JM. Glomerulocystic kidney disease and hemolytic-uremic síndrome: clinicopathological case. *Nefrologia.* 2000; 20(5): 459-63.

[48]   Amir G., Rosenmann E., Drukker A. Adquiredglomerulocystic kidney disease following hemolytic-uremic síndrome. *Pediat. Nephrol.* 1995; 9(5): 614-16.

[49]   Obata Y., Furusu A., Miyazaki M., Nishino T., Kawazu T., Kanamoto Y. et al. Glomerulocystic kidney disease in an adult with enlarged kidneys: a case report and review of the literatura. *Clin. Nephrol.* 2011; 75(2): 158-64.

[50]   Gupta K., Vankalakunti M., Sachdeva MU. Glomerulocystic kidney disease and its rare associations: an autopsy report of two unrelated cases. *Diagn. Pathol.* 2007; 25: 2-12.

[51]   Lima E., La Fuente J., García Cuerpo E., Sánchez Encinas M., Fernández González I., SánzMigueláñez JL. Et al.Pyelocalycealdiverticula. *Arch. Esp. Urol.* 2000; 53(7):

[52]   581-95.

[53]   Matlaga BR., Miller NL., Terry C., Kim SC., Kuo RL., Coe FL. et al. The pathogenesis of calyceal diverticular calculi. *Urol. Res.* 2007, 35(1): 35-40.

[54]   Garrido Abad P., Fernández González I., Coloma del Peso A., Herranz Fernández LM., Jiménez Gálvez M., Fernández Arjona M. et al. Percutaneous treatment of calyceal diverticulum associated with lithiasis. *Arch. Esp. Urol.* 2009; 62(1): 42-48.

[55]   Stunell H., McNeill G., Brown RF., Granger R., Torreggiani WC. The imaging appearances of calyceal diverticula complicated by urolithiasis. *Br. J. Radiol.* 2010, 83(994): 888-94.

[56]   Eble JN., Sauter G., Epstein J., Sesterhenn A., editors. Tumours of the Urinary System and Male Genital Organs. Pathology and Genetics. WHO Classification of Tumours. IARC 2004. Lyon.

[57]   Moch H. Cystic renal tumors: new entities and novel concepts. *Adv. Anat. Pathol.* 2010, 17(3): 209-14.

[58]   Eble JN., Bonsib SM. Extensively cystic renal neoplasms: cystic nephroma, cystic partially differentiated nephroblastoma, multilocular cystic renal cell carcinoma and cystic hamartoma of renal pelvis. *Semin. Diagn. Pathol.* 1988; 15(1): 2-20.

[59]   Zhou M., Kort E., Hoekstra P., Westphal M., Magi-Galluzzi C., Sercia L. et al. Adult cystic nephroma and mixed epitelial and stromal tumor of the kidney are the same

didease entity: molecular and histologic evidence. *Am. J. Surg. Pathol.* 2009; 33: 72-80.

[60]   Turbiner J., Amin MB., Humphrey PA., Srigley JR., De Leval L., Radhakrishnan A. et al. Cystic nephroma and mixed epithelial and stromal tumor of kidney: a detailed clinicopathologic analysis of 34 cases and proposal for renal epithelial and stromal tumor (REST) as a unifying term. *Am. J. Surg. Pathol.* 2007; 31: 489-500.

[61]   Castaño JC., Velez A., RaulFlorez F., Uribe CA. Renal lymphangioma. *Arch. Esp. Urol.* 2005; 58(3): 256-58.

[62]   Honma I., Takagi Y., Shigyo M., Sunaoshi K., Wakabayashi J., Harada O. et al. Lymphangioma of thekidney. *Int. J. Urol.* 2002; 9(3): 178-82.

[63]   Bagheri MH., Zare Z., Sefidbakht S., Nabavizadeh SA., Meshksar A., RoozbehJ., et al. Bilateral renal lymphangiomatosis: sonographic findings. *J. Clin. Ultrasound.* 2009; 37(2): 115-18.

[64]   Murad T., Komaiko W., Oyasu R., Bauer K. Multilocular cystic renal cell carcinoma. *Am. J. Clin. Pathol.* 1991; 95: 633-637.

[65]   Brinker DA., Amin MB., de Peralta- Venturine M., Reuter VG., Chan TY., Epstein JI. Extensively necrotic cystic renal cell carcinoma: a clinicopathologic study with comparison to other cystic and necrotic renal cancers. *Am. J. Surg. Pathol.* 2000; 24: 988-95.

[66]   Mac Lennan GT., Ross J., Cheng L. Cystic partially differentiated nephroblastoma. *J. Urol.* 2010; 183(4): 1585-86.

[67]   Nagao T., Sugano I., Ishida Y., Tajima Y., Masai M., Nagakura K. et al. Cystic partially differentiated nephroblastoma in an adult: an immunohistochemical, lectinhistochemical and ultrastuctural study. *Histopathology* 1999; 35: 65-73.

[68]   Van den Hoek., de Krijger R., van de Venk, Lequin M., van den Heuvel-Eibrink MM. Cystic nephroma, cystic partially differentiated nephroblastoma and cystic Wilm's tumor in children: a spectrum with therapeutic dilemmas. *Urol. Int.* 2009; 82(1): 65-70.

[69]   Momohara C., Komori K., Takada T., Imazu T., Honda M., Fujioka H. A case of renalangiomyolipoma with marked cystic degeneration and pseudoaneurysm. *Hinyokik Kiyo.* 2002 Feb; 48(2):105-8.

[70]   Adenoma metanéfrico renal de predominio quístico. A propósito de un caso. Torres Gómez FJ., García Escudero A., Torres Olivera FJ. *Arch. Esp. Urol.* 2006; 59(1):

[71]   90-92.

[72]   Kodama K., Nagano K., Akimoto M., Suzuki S. Small renaloncocytoma with central cystic degeneration. *Int. J. Urol.* 2004 Feb; 11(2):110-3.

[73]   Osako Y., Tatarano S., Nishiyama K., Yamada Y., Yamagata T., Uchida Y., Nakagawa M. Unusual presentation of intraparenchymalrenal artery aneurysm mimicking cysticrenal cell carcinoma: a case report. *Int. J. Urol.* 2011 Jul; 18(7): 533-5. doi: 10.1111/j.1442-2042.2011.02775.x. Epub 2011 May 16.

[74]   Bosniak MA. The current radiologic approach to renal cysts. *Radiology* 1986;158:1-0.

[75]   Hartman DS., Davis CJ., Johns T., Goldman SM. Cystic renal cell carcinoma. *Urology* 1986;28: 145–153.

[76]   Bosniak MA. Diagnosis and management of patients with complicated cystic lesions of the kidney. *AJR.* 1997;169: 819–821.

[77] Uppot RN., Harisinghani, Gervais DA. Imaging-Guided Percutaneous Renal Biopsy: *Rationale and Approach Am. J. Roentgenol.* June 1, 2010 194:1443-1449.

[78] Harisinghani MG., Maher MM., Gervais DA. et al. Incidence of malignancy in complex cystic renal masses (Bosniak category III): should imaging-guided biopsy precede surgery? *AJR* 2003 ;180: 755 –758.

[79] Whelan TF. Guidelines on the management of renal cyst disease. *Can. Urol. Assoc. J.* 2010 April; 4(2): 98–99.

[80] Israel GM., Bosniak MA. Calcification in cystic renal masses: Is it important in diagnosis? *Radiology.* 2003;226:47–52.

[81] Curry NS., Cochran ST., Bissada NK. Cystic renal masses: accurate Bosniak classification requires adequate renal CT. *AJR. Am. J. Roentgenol.* 2000;175:339–42.

[82] Touloupidis S. et al. Percutaneous drainage of simple cysts of the kidney: a new method. *Urol. Int.* 2004;73(2):169-72.

[83] Akinci D. et al. Long-term results of single-session percutaneous drainage and ethanol sclerotherapy in simple renal cysts. *Eur. J. Radiol.* 2005 May; 54(2):298-302.

[84] Nadu A., Ekstein P., Szold A., Friedman A., Nakache R., Cohen Y. et al. Ventilatory and hemodynamic changes during retroperitoneal and transperitoneal laparoscopic nephrectomy: a prospective real-time comparison. *J. Urol.* Sep 2005;174(3):1013-7.

[85] Soderdahl DW. and Fabrizio MD. Laparoscopic Evaluation and Treatment of Symptomatic and Indeterminate Renal Cysts. In: Atlas of Laparoscopic Urologic Surgery. Michigan University. Saunders/Elsevier Eds: 2008.

[86] Desai MM. et al. Scarless single port transumbilical nephrectomy and pyeloplasty: first clinical report. *BJU Int.* 2008; 101: 83-88.

[87] Santos BF. and Hungness ES. Natural orifice translumenal endoscopic surgery: Progress in humans since white paper. *World J. Gastroenterol.* 2011 April 7; 17(13): 1655-1665.

[88] Sotelo R., de Andrade R., Fernández G., Ramirez D., Di Grazia E. Carmona O., Moreira O., Berger A., Aron M., Desai MM., Gill IS. NOTES hybrid transvaginal radical nephrectomy for tumor: stepwise progression toward a first successful clinical case. *Eur. Urol.* 2010;57:138-144.

[89] Lehmann KS., Ritz JP., Wibmer A., Gellert K., Zornig C., Burghardt J., Büsing M., Runkel N., Kohlhaw K., Albrecht R. The German registry for natural orifice translumenal endoscopic surgery: report of the first 551 patients. *Ann. Surg.* 2010;252:263-270.

[90] Roy S., Dillon MJ., Trompeter RS., Barratt TM. Autosomal recessive polycystic kidney disease: long-term outcome of neonatal survivors. *Pediatr. Nephrol.* 1997;11:302–6.

[91] Guay-Woodford LM., Desmond RA. Autosomal recessive polycystic kidney disease: the clinical experience in North America. *Pediatrics.* 2003;111:1072–80.

[92] Bergmann C. et al. Clinical consequences of PKHD1 mutations in 164 patients with autosomal-recessive polycystic kidney disease (ARPKD). *Kidney Int.* 2005;67:829–48.

[93] Zeier M. et al. Renal histology in polycystic kidney disease with incipient and advanced renal failure. *Kidney Int.* 1992;42:1259-65.

[94] Bello-Reuss E. et al. Angiogenesis in autosomal-dominant polycystic kidney disease. *Kidney Int.* 2001;60:37-45.

[95] Wilson PD. Polycystic Kidney Disease. *N. Engl. J. Med.* 2004;350: 151-64.

[96] Jafar TH. et al. The effect of angiotensin-converting-enzyme inhibitors on progression of advanced polycystic kidney disease. *Kidney Int.* 2005;67:265-71.

[97] Cadnapaphornchai MA. et al. Design and baseline characteristics of participants in the study of antihypertensive therapy in children and adults with autosomal dominant polycystic kidney disease (ADPKD). *Contemp. Clin. Trials* 2005;26:211-22.

[98] Ecder T. et al. Diuretic versus angiotensin-converting enzyme inhibitors in autosomal dominant polycystic kidney disease. *Am. J. Nephrol.* 2001;21:98-103.

[99] Cases A. and Coll E. Dyslipidemia and the progression of renal disease in chronic renal failure patients. *Kidney Int.* 2005;68 Suppl. 99:S87-93.

[100] Torres VE. et al. Effective treatment of an orthologous model of autosomal dominant polycystic kidney disease. *Nature Med.* 2004;10:363-4.

[101] Van Dijk MA. et al. Effect of simvastatin on renal function in autosomal polycystic kidney disease. *Nephrol. Dial Transplant.* 2001;16:2152-7.

[102] Cowley BD. et al. Elevated c-mycprotooncogene expression in autosomal recessive polycystic kidney disease. *Proc. Natl. Acad. Sci.* US 1988;85:2578.

[103] Harding MA. et al. Localization of overexpressed c-myc mRNA in polycystic kidneys of the cpk mouse. *Kidney Int.*1992;41:317-25.

[104] Husson H. et al. New insights into ADPKD molecular pathways using combination of SAGE and microarray technologies. *Genomics* 2004;84:497-510.

[105] Trudel M. et al. C-myc as an inducer of polycystic disease in transgenic mice. *Kidney Int.*1991;39:665-71.

[106] Ricker JL. et al. Development of autosomal recessive polycystic kidney disease in BALB/c-cpk/cpk mice. *J. Am. Soc. Nephrol.* 2000;11:1837-47.

[107] Gattone VH. Emerging therapies for polycystic kidney disease. *Curr. Opinion Pharm.* 2005;5:535-42.

[108] Fingar DC., Blenis J. Target of rapamycin (TOR): An integrator of nutrient and growth factor signals and coordinator of cell growth and cell cycle progression. *Oncogene* 2004; 23: 3151–3171.

[109] Kim DH. et al: mTOR interacts with raptor to form a nutrient-sensitive complex that signals to the cell growth machinery. *Cell* 2002; 110: 163–175.

[110] Berthier CC. et al. Sirolimus ameliorates the enhanced expression of metalloproteinases in a rat model of autosomal dominant polycystic kidney disease. *Nephrol. Dial Transplant.* 2008;23: 880–889.

[111] Perico N. et al. Sirolimustherapyto halt the progression of ADPKD. *J. Am. Soc. Nephrol.* 2010; 21(6): 1031–1040.

[112] Ruggenenti P. et al. Safety and efficacy of long-acting somatostatin treatment in autosomal-dominant polycystic kidney disease. *Kidney Int.* 2005;68:206-16.

[113] Hogan MC. et al. Randomized Clinical Trial of Long-Acting Somatostatin for Autosomal Dominant Polycystic Kidney and Liver Disease. *J. Am. Soc. Nephrol.* 2010;21(6):1052-61.

[114] Gattone VH. et al.Inhibition of renal cystic disease development and progression by a vasopressin V2 receptor antagonist. *Nature Med.* 2003; 9:1323-6.

[115] Calvet JP. Strategies to inhibit cyst formation in ADPKD. *Clin. J. Am. Soc. Nephrol.* 2008; 3: 1205–1211.

[116] TorresVE. et al. Effective treatment of an orthologous model of autosomal dominant polycystic kidney disease. *Nature Med.* 2004;10:363-4.

[117] Torres VE. Role of vasopressin antagonists. *Clin. J. Am. Soc. Nephrol.* 2008; 3:1212–1218.

In: Cysts: Causes, Diagnosis and Treatment Options
Editors: A. Mendes Ortiz and A. Jimenez Moreno

ISBN: 978-1-62081-315-7
© 2012 Nova Science Publishers, Inc.

Chapter 4

CYSTS: CAUSES, DIAGNOSIS AND TREATMENT OPTIONS

Inmaculada Oller Navarro, *Jaime Ruiz-Tovar Polo* *and Rafael Calpena Rico*

Hospital General Universitario de Elche, Alicante, Spain

INTRODUCTION

Cystic lesions of the liver represent a heterogeneous group of disorders, which differ in etiology, prevalence, and clinical manifestations.

The term liver cyst usually refers to solitary nonparasitic cysts, also known as simple cysts. However, several other cystic lesions must be distinguished from true simple cysts. Cystic lesions of the liver include simple cysts, multiple cysts arising in the setting of polycystic liver disease (PCLD), parasitic or hydatid (echinococcal) cysts, cystic tumors, and abscesses (1-3).

The precise frequency of liver cysts is not known because most are asymptomatic, but liver cysts have been estimated to occur in 5% of the population. No more than 10-15% of these patients have symptoms that bring the cyst to clinical attention. Liver cysts are usually found as an incidental finding on imaging or at the time of laparotomy. Most series in the literature are relatively small, reporting fewer than 50 patients each. Furthermore, consensus has not been achieved on the optimal treatment of patients with symptomatic cysts, although a number of therapeutic approaches have been described (5,6).

This topic review will provide an overview of the causes, diagnosis and management of cystic lesions in the liver.

*Address for Correspondence: Hospital General Universitario De El Che, Camino De La Almazara, 11.03203 El Che Alicante Espana, -e-mail: inma-oller@hotmail.com, -TLF; (0034) 645204961

1. SIMPLE CYSTS

Etiopathology

The cause of simple liver cysts is unknown, but they are believed to be congenital in origin. The cysts are lined by biliary-type epithelium and perhaps result from progressive dilation of biliary microhamartomas. Because these cysts seldom contain bile, the current hypothesis is that the microhamartomas fail to develop normal connections with the biliary tree. Typically, the fluid within the cyst has an electrolyte composition that mimics plasma. Bile, amylase, and white blood cells are absent. The cyst fluid is continually secreted by the epithelial lining of the cyst. For this reason, needle aspiration of simple cysts is not curative.

Epidemiology

Although simple cysts are found in approximately 1% of necropsied adults, very few become large, and even fewer cause symptoms. Their size ranges from a few millimeters to massive lesions occupying large volumes of the upper abdomen; the largest reported cyst contained 17 liters of fluid (7).

Simple cysts tend to occur more commonly in the right lobe, and are more prevalent in women. The female-to-male ratio is approximately 1.5:1 among those with asymptomatic simple cysts while it is 9:1 in those with symptomatic or complicated simple cysts (1). Huge cysts are found almost exclusively in women over 50.

Clinical Manifestations

Symptomatic patients may present with abdominal discomfort, pain, or nausea. As a general rule, cysts in symptomatic patients are larger than those in asymptomatic ones(6,8). Large cysts can produce atrophy of the adjacent hepatic tissue while huge cysts can cause complete atrophy of a hepatic lobe with compensatory hypertrophy of the other lobe. Occasionally, a cyst is large enough to produce a palpable abdominal mass. Jaundice caused by bile duct obstruction is rare, as well as cyst rupture and acute torsion of a mobile cyst. Patients with cyst torsion may present with an acute abdomen. When simple cysts rupture, patients may develop secondary infection, leading to a presentation similar to a hepatic abscess with abdominal pain, fever, and leukocytosis.(2-4)

Diagnosis

The distinction between a simple cyst, cystadenoma, cystadenocarcinoma, echinococcal cyst and other rare primary or metastatic tumors can be difficult. However, the distinction is extremely important since these lesions have different clinical significance (Table 1).

Table 1. Clinical manifestation and imaging findings pointing against the diagnosis of a simple cyst

Manifestatinon/imaging findings	Differential diagnosis
Progressive symptoms	Cystadenoma,cystadenocarcinoma,metastasis.
Abnormal hepatic biochemical test	Cystadenocarcinoma,metastasis.
Rapid growth on periodic follow-up	Cystadenoma,cystadenocarcinoma,metastasis.
Calcification on daughter cysts	Echinococcal cysts
Thick or irregular cyst wall	Cystadenoma,cystadenocarcinoma,metastasis, Echinococcal cysts.
Nonhomogeneus cyst content	Cystadenoma,cystadenocarcinoma, Echinococcal cysts,bleeding into a simple cyst.
Sepations or multilocular cyst space.	Cystadenoma,cystadenocarcinoma, Echinococcal cysts,bleeding into a simple cyst.

- Imaging studies

Ultrasonography is probably the most helpful initial test since it can usually differentiate a simple cyst from other cystic lesions. It should also be used for follow-up studies. Simple cysts appear as an anechoic unilocular fluid filled space with imperceptible walls, and with posterior acoustic enhancement (9). Clinical features combined with the sonographic findings are usually sufficient to distinguish simple cysts from other lesions that can appear cystic such as a liver abscess, necrotic malignant tumor, hemangioma, and hamartoma.

On a CT scan a simple cyst is defined as a well-demarcated water attenuation lesion that does not enhance following the administration of intravenous contrast. Uncomplicated simple cysts are virtually never septated. However, hemorrhage into a simple cyst can lead to confusion in the sonographic differentiation from a cystadenoma or cystadenocarcinoma (4,10). In one report, hemorrhage was associated with the appearance of septa in 2 of 57 patients (3.5 percent) with large simple cysts (≥4 cm) (11). Hemorrhage is much less frequent in smaller cysts.

Magnetic resonance imaging (MRI) demonstrates a well-defined water-attenuation lesion that does not enhance following the administration of intravenous Gadolinium. On T1-weighted images the cyst shows a low signal, whereas a very high intensity signal is shown on T2-weighted images.

Differential Diagnosis

The differential diagnosis of a simple cyst includes a variety of liver lesions that can have a cystic appearance, such as cystadenoma, cystadenocarcinoma, hepatic abscess, a necrotic malignant tumor, hemangioma, and hamartoma. As mentioned above, the distinction can usually be made based upon the clinical setting and radiographic findings. A rare exception is a hepatic metastasis from a neuroendocrine tumor, which can be asymptomatic and can have a sharply-defined necrotic area. (Table 2).

Table 2. Differential diagnosis in imaging studies

	US	CT	MRI
Simple cyst	-anechoic unilocular fluid filled space -thin walls -posterior acoustic enhancement [	-anechoic unilocular fluid filled space -imperceptible walls -posterior acoustic enhancement -non septated	-well-defined water-attenuation lesion -not contrast enhanced
Cystadenoma	-hypoechoic lesion -thickened irregular walls -occasional internal echoes	-low attenuated mass -uni- or multilocular -septations -thickened and/or irregular wall	-low attenuated mass -uni- or multilocular -septations -thickened and/or irregular wall
Cystadeno-carcinoma	-Multilocular -Irregular walls	-Similar to cystadenomas	-Similar to cystadenomas
Hydatid cyst	-liver cyst contains membranes -mixed echoes -reveals infoldings of the inner cyst wall, separation of the hydatid membrane from the wall of the cyst, or hydatid sand.	-hydatid sand, daughter cysts, and splitting of the cyst wall. -detecting gas and minute calcifications within the cysts.	-has no major advantage over CT.
Biliary cyst	-often the first imaging modality used -may show a cystic mass in the right upper quadrant -has no major advantage over CT.	-can detect all types of biliary cysts. -can demonstrate continuity of the cyst with the biliary tree. -examine the relationship to surrounding structures, and can evaluate for the presence of malignancy	-show dilated portion of the bile duct or ampulla. -Cholangiography can identify an abnormal pancreatobiliary junction, and can detect filling defects due to stones or malignancy. -Magnetic resonance cholangiopancreatography (MRCP) does not have the risks of cholangitis and pancreatitis associated with direct cholangiography, and in many cases it is the test of choice for diagnosing.

Histopathology

Histological examination is seldom needed for establishing the diagnosis. However, when histology is available, the following criteria can be used for a definitive diagnosis:

- An outer layer of a thin dense fibrous tissue
- An inner epithelial lining consisting of a single layer of cuboidal or columnar epithelium; this layer is found in most but not in all simple cysts
- Lack of mesenchymal stroma or cellular atypia

Treatment

The majority of simple cysts do not require treatment. However, it may be prudent to monitor large cysts (≥4 cm in diameter) periodically with ultrasonography to assure that they remain stable. We suggest an initial follow-up study in 3 months after the diagnosis and then again at 6 to 12 months. Further monitoring is usually unnecessary if the cyst remains unchanged for two to three years.

The presence of symptoms related to the cyst or increasing size should raise concern that the lesion could be a cystadenoma, a cystadenocarcinoma, or another rare cystic neoplasm, since simple cysts tend to remain stable in size. Such patients may require surgical intervention. The causal relationship between abdominal pain or discomfort and a simple cyst must be admitted with caution, and accepted only if the cyst is large, and other possible causes of the symptoms have been excluded. These include cholelithiasis, gastroesophageal reflux disease, gastric dysmotility, peptic ulcer disease, and other causes of dyspepsia. Percutaneous aspiration has been advocated as a diagnostic test for relief of symptoms (12). However, this test is not without risk, and has not been widely accepted. Several therapeutic approaches have been described for symptomatic, large simple cysts including needle aspiration with or without injection of sclerosing agents (13), internal drainage with cystojejunostomy (14), wide unroofing (15,16), and varying degrees of liver resection. In most series, percutaneous needle aspiration was associated with a high failure rate and rapid recurrence .Percutaneous needle aspiration with injection of sclerosing agents is generally safe, effective, and relatively non-invasive (18,19); however, it may occasionally have serious complications (20). Wide unroofing or cyst resection has been associated with a relatively low incidence of cyst recurrence or complications (11,15,16,21). The laparoscopic approach has proven to be safe, achieving a wide unroofing or resection without the need for a debilitating incision (11,16,21,22).

Several centers have reported recurrence rates ranging from 0 - 14.3% and morbidity rates of 0-15% after laparoscopic unroofing of solitary simple cysts (16,23). Potential complications of laparoscopic unroofing include wound infection, bile leak, subphrenic hematoma, and prolonged serosal postoperative discharge through abdominal drain (>3 days) (16) Laparoscopic unroofing may not be possible in patients with a superior or posterior location of the cyst. There are no prospective studies comparing the different therapeutic approaches. As a result the procedure of choice should be decided on a case by case basis, taking into consideration the cyst's location, suspicion of malignancy, history of abdominal surgery, and local expertise.

2. CYSTADENOMA

Hepatobiliary cystadenomas are rare cystic tumours that occur within the liver parenchyma or, less frequently, in the extrahepatic bile ducts. The published experience with these lesions is limited to single case reports and small series (11,26,27). These reports suggest that cystadenomas occur in adults, more often in women. The tumours usually appear more frequently in the right lobe than in the left one, but some series have reported frequent involvement of the left lobe.The tumours grew to a large size and required surgical intervention in most series.

Clinical Manifestations

The most commonly reported presenting symptoms were a sensation of an upper abdominal mass, abdominal discomfort or pain, and anorexia. These symptoms had been present for several years prior to diagnosis in several patients. However, many patients were asymptomatic, and the lesions were found incidentally on abdominal imaging studies.

Diagnosis

Histologic examination is required for definitive diagnosis, although the lesion may be suspected on imaging studies. The differential diagnosis includes cystadenocarcinoma, echinococcal cyst, and a simple cyst. Simple cysts can usually be distinguished because of the absence of septations and papillary projections and the presence of serous cystic fluid. Echinococcal cysts are frequently associated with calcifications and patients will have positive serology.

- Imaging studies

The appearance of cystadenoma on ultrasonography can usually differentiate it from a simple cyst .On ultrasonography, a cystadenoma typically appears as an hypoechoic lesion with thickened irregular walls and occasional internal echoes representing debris and wall nodularity. These findings are generally indicative of a complicated cyst, which may represent a simple cyst with previous bleeding, a neoplastic cyst such as a cystadenoma, cystadenocarcinoma, or rarely a metastasis. On a CT scan a cystadenoma appears as a low attenuated mass, which may be uni- or multilocular, or may have septations .The cyst wall is usually thickened and/or irregular. This is in contrast to a simple cyst, which is typically devoid of septations and has imperceptible walls.

Histopathology

A cystadenoma is usually a multilocular cystic lesion with a smooth external surface, and a thin wall with smooth internal lining. The cyst frequently contains blood or browned-coloured material. Histology is essential for the diagnosis and is usually obtained during or after resection of a suspicious cyst. Microscopically, cystadenomas are lined by biliary type mucus-secreting cuboidal or columnar epithelium, supported by dense cellular (mesenchymal) fibrous stroma resembling ovarian tissue. The lining is surrounded by a loose and less cellular layer of collagen. It has been suggested that hepatobiliary cystadenoma may be composed of two distinct groups that differ in the presence or absence of a mesenchymal stroma surrounding the epithelial lining of the cyst (25).

Treatment. The preferred treatment for cystadenomas is surgical resection, which should be performed whenever possible since malignant transformation of the cyst lining has been described in as many as 15% of patients (27). Removal of the cyst can be accomplished by enucleating it from the surrounding liver. Partial excision is invariably associated with recurrence and with worse prognosis compared to complete resection (16). Aspiration is also associated with rapid recurrence of fluid and symptoms (11). A hepatic resection should be considered whenever a cystic lesion is suspected of being a cystadenocarcinoma since reliable differentiation between cystadenoma and cystadenocarcinoma is not always possible (28).

3. CYSTADENOCARCINOMA

Cystadenocarcinomas probably arise from malignant transformation of a cystadenoma. This tumor is usually found in the elderly, although it has been reported in patients in their thirties. While the tumors can invade adjacent tissues and metastasize, their prognosis has generally been better than that associated with cholangiocarcinoma (24).

Diagnosis

The distinction between a cystadenoma and cystadenocarcinoma can be difficult to make based upon clinical, radiologic, and histological evidence (28,29). Cystadenocarcinomas are usually multilocular and resemble cystadenomas. Malignant changes are typically found in the inner epithelial lining.

Histopathology

Macroscopically, cystadenoma, and cystadenocarcinomas have a smooth external surface. However, internally, cystadenomas have varying degrees of thickness in the wall, although infrequently they may have a thin wall with a smooth lining. Cystadenocarcinomas generally have a thick wall that may show large tissue masses protruding from the internal cyst lining (24,25). Cystadenocarcinomas have occasionally been identified preoperatively by aspiration and examination of the contents of the cyst, but this procedure carries a risk of bleeding and peritoneal seeding of the tumor (30). As noted above, elevated levels of CEA have been reported in cystic fluid aspirated from a cystadenocarcinoma, but the diagnostic accuracy of this finding is not clear.

Treatment

In contrast to a cystadenoma, if cystadenocarcinoma is suspected, treatment should consist of a formal liver resection (28,31). Enucleation is not recommended since it may be associated with an increased risk of recurrence. The lesion is potentially curable by complete excision. The effect of nonsurgical therapy (eg, radiation or chemotherapy) is unknown.

4. ECHINOCOCCAL CYSTS

Etiopathology

Echinococcal (hydatid) cysts of the liver are caused by the larval form of *Echinococcus granulosus*, which is usually acquired from infected dogs. These are fluid-filled structures limited by a parasite-derived membrane, which contains germinal epithelium. Four species of Echinococcus produce infection in humans; *E. granulosus and E. multilocularis* are the most common ones, causing cystic echinococcosis (CE) and alveolar echinococcosis (AE), respectively. The two other species, *E. vogeli and E. oligarthus*, cause polycystic echinococcosis but have only rarely been associated with human infection.

Clinical Manifestations

Patients are often asymptomatic. When symptoms appear, they are usually due to the mass effect of an enlarging cyst or complications such as intraperitoneal leakage, infection, or biliary obstruction. *E. granulosus* cysts can rupture into the biliary tree and produce biliary colic, obstructive jaundice, cholangitis, or pancreatitis. Pressure or mass effects on the bile ducts, portal and hepatic veins, or on the inferior vena cava can result in cholestasis, portal hypertension, venous obstruction, or the Budd-Chiari syndrome.

Liver cysts can also rupture into the peritoneum causing peritonitis, or transdiaphragmatically into the bronchial tree causing pulmonary hydatidosis or a bronchial fistula. Secondary bacterial infection of the cysts can result in liver abscesses.

Diagnosis

The combination of imaging and serology usually make the diagnosis of cystic echinococcosis (71), although serologic assays are more sensitive and specific for *E. multilocularis* compared to *E. granulosus* infection.

- Routinary laboratory tests:

Nonspecific leukopenia or thrombocytopenia, mild eosinophilia, and nonspecific liver function abnormalities may be detected, but are not diagnostic. Fewer than 15 percent of cases have eosinophilia, which generally occurs only if there is leakage of antigenic material.

- Imaging studies

Ultrasound has a sensitivity of approximately 90-95% (13,14). The most common appearance on ultrasound is an anechoic smooth, round cyst, which can be difficult to distinguish from a benign cyst. When the liver cyst contains membranes, mixed echoes will appear that can be confused with an abscess or neoplasm. When daughter cysts are present, characteristic internal septation results. Ultrasound allows for the classification of the cysts by biologic activity, which may influence the choice of treatment; these categories are: active, transitional, or inactive. Characteristics on ultrasound that are suggestive of an inactive lesion include a collapsing, flattened elliptical cyst (corresponds to low pressure within the cyst), detachment of the germinal layer from the cyst wall ("water lily sign"), coarse echoes within the cyst, and calcification of the cyst wall (16,17). Cysts with a calcified rim may have an "eggshell" appearance.

Computed tomography. Many reports suggest that CT has a higher overall sensitivity than ultrasound, with sensitivity rates of 95-100% (13,14,16). CT is the best mode for determining the number, size, and anatomic location of the cysts, and is also better than ultrasound in detecting extrahepatic cysts. CT may also be used for monitoring lesions during therapy and to detect recurrences (21). CT may be superior to ultrasound in determining complications such as infection and intrabiliary rupture (22).

Magnetic resonance imaging .MRI has no major advantage over CT for abdominal or pulmonary hydatid cysts, except in defining changes in the intra- and extrahepatic venous system (24). However, it may delineate the cyst capsule better than CT and may be better at diagnosing complications, particularly for cysts with infection or biliary communication. Both MRI and CT are useful in diagnosing echinococcal infection in other sites, such as in the brain(28).

- Serology

Immunodiagnosis is useful for primary diagnosis and for follow-up after treatment (8,29,30). Detection of circulating *E. granulosus* antigens in serum is less sensitive than antibody detection, which remains the method of choice (8).

Conventional routine immunodiagnostic tests are usually based upon the use of crude antigens, such as hydatid fluid or protoscolex extracts. Additional tests using recombinant or purified species-specific antigens may complement the serological diagnosis (31).

Serologic testing produces both many false positive and false negative results.

- False positive reactions are more likely in the presence of other helminth infections (such as *Taenia saginata, Taenia solium*, and particularly neurocysticercosis), cancer, and immune disorders.

- False negative results occur with varying frequency depending upon the site of the lesion and the cyst's integrity and viability. Antigen-antibody complexes that "mop" up all antibodies may lead to false negative reactions. Thus, a negative serologic test generally does not rule out echinococcosis.

Children and pregnant women more frequently have negative serology than other patient populations(2).

The methods most frequently employed for initial screening tests (using crude antigens) are Indirect hemagglutination (IHA) and Enzyme-linked immunosorbent assay (ELISA). Confirmatory tests using specific antigens can then be performed, such as arc-5 immunoelectrophoresis and immunoblotting (34).

- Cyst aspiration or biopsy

Percutaneous aspiration or biopsy may be required to confirm the diagnosis by demonstrating the presence of protoscolices, hooklets, or hydatid membranes. Active cysts reveal clear watery fluid containing scolices and have elevated pressure, whereas inactive cysts exhibit cloudy fluid without detectable scolices and do not have elevated pressure(16).

Percutaneous aspiration of liver cyst contents is associated with very low rates of complications, but this method of diagnosis is generally reserved for situations when other diagnostic methods are inconclusive because of the potential for anaphylaxis and secondary spread of the infection(62). If aspiration is required, it should be performed under ultrasound or CT guidance; complications can be minimized by concurrent administration of benzimidazole therapy.

Treatment

In the past, open surgery was the only option for the treatment of echinococcal cysts. However, experience is increasing with other potential treatment modalities, including laparoscopic techniques, the PAIR (Percutaneous Aspiration, Introduction of a protoscolicidal agent, and Reaspiration) procedure(43), and chemotherapy, which in certain cases renders open techniques unnecessary (1).

Actually, surgery is being reserved for those patients in whom percutaneous treatment is not available. However, open surgery remains the first treatment choice for complicated cysts, and it is also an option for complete removal of the parasite in patients who can tolerate surgery and who have cysts in amenable locations. Surgery is generally the preferred option for large liver cysts (diameter >10 cm, especially if associated with multiple daughter cysts); superficially located single liver cysts that have a risk of rupture; complicated cysts such as those accompanied by infection, compression, or obstruction; or cysts in the lung, kidney, bone, brain, or other organs (34,36-38).

According to the WHO (World Health Organisation) informal working group panel, indications for surgery for liver echinococcosis include (35):

- Removal of large developing and transitional cysts with multiple daughter vesicles.
- Single liver cysts situated superficially that may rupture spontaneously or as a result of trauma. Open surgery should be considered if percutaneous treatment is not available .
- Infected cysts when percutaneous treatment is not amenable .
- As an alternative to percutaneous therapy for cysts communicating with the biliary tree .
- Management of cysts exerting pressure on adjacent vital organs.

Surgery is contraindicated in:

- Patients for whom general contraindications for surgery apply, such as those whose general condition is very poor
- Patients with multiple cysts or cysts that are difficult to access
- Patients with inactive, totally calcified asymptomatic cysts
- Patients with very small cysts

- Adjunctive chemotherapy

Adjunctive chemotherapy (usually with albendazole or mebendazole) before and after surgery appears to reduce the risk of recurrence, by inactivating protoscolices and reducing cyst tension for easier removal (39). If spillage of cyst contents occurs spontaneously or following manipulation, albendazole or mebendazole should be continued to reduce the risk of secondary hydatidosis. Many would also administer a course of praziquantel in this situation (one to seven days). The optimal duration of chemotherapy before and after surgical procedures is uncertain.

Therapy generally should be begun at least four days before surgery (the WHO informal working group recommends between four days and one month) and be continued for at least one month (albendazole) or three months (mebendazole) following surgery.

- Percutaneous treatments

Percutaneous treatments can broadly be divided into: (1) those aiming at the destruction of the germinal layer (puncture, aspiration, injection and reaspiration, or PAIR) and (2) those aiming at the evacuation of the entire endocyst (also known as Modified Catheterization Techniques). Percutaneous drainage is gaining acceptance because of its low morbidity and easy applicability, but the patient selection is of paramount importance (34).

- PAIR procedure: Puncture, aspiration, injection and reaspiration (PAIR) is a percutaneous cyst puncture procedure performed under ultrasound or CT guidance followed by aspiration of substantial amounts of cyst fluid and injection of a protoscolicidal agent into the cyst cavity (usually hypertonic saline or ethanol). The cyst is then reaspirated after a period of at least 15 minutes. The development of fine needles and catheters, the advances in imaging techniques, and the introduction of the intercostal intrahepatic approach, minimizes the risk of anaphylactic shock or spillage associated with PAIR. PAIR has increasingly become the treatment of choice in many situations (40). PAIR has the benefits of confirming the diagnosis and removing parasitic material, but is minimally invasive, less risky and usually less expensive than open surgery (41). Safety is based on data from more than 4000 PAIR procedures over more than 20 years (35).

- Indications and contraindications .PAIR has been used largely for cysts in the liver and other abdominal locations (eg, abdominal cavity, spleen, kidney). Cysts in other sites (eg, bone and lung) occasionally have been treated in this fashion, but complications and failures have been observed more frequently in these cases.

- PAIR is warranted for patients at high surgical risk, those who refuse surgery, pregnant patients, and in cases of relapse after surgery or failure to respond to medical therapy alone. PAIR is indicated for uncomplicated simple hydatid cysts filled with clear fluid, with or without a detached membrane or daughter cysts. However, PAIR should not be performed in patients with inaccessible cysts, superficially located liver cysts where there is a risk of spillage into the abdominal cavity, cysts with nondrainable solid material or echogenic foci, inactive or calcified cysts, cysts that have ruptured into the biliary system or peritoneum, or cysts with biliary communication (38).

- Treatment with albendazole for a minimum of 4 hours before PAIR and for one month following PAIR should be administered (34,42).

5. OTHER CYSTIC LESIONS OF THE LIVER

A variety of other cystic lesions of the liver have been described the clinical significance of which are variable.

- Ciliated hepatic foregut cyst

A ciliated foregut cyst is a rare, benign solitary cyst consisting of ciliated pseudostratified columnar epithelium, subepithelial connective tissue, a smooth muscle layer, and an outer fibrous capsule. Unlike simple solitary cysts, they occur more frequently in men, and are found most commonly in the left lobe (32).

There are about 60 reported cases of ciliated foregut cyst, the size of which ranged from 0.4 to 9.0 cm. There are no reported cases of malignant transformation. The clinical importance of its diagnosis lies in the distinction from other potentially malignant hepatic lesions.

- Primary squamous cell carcinoma

There are several reports of primary squamous cell carcinoma arising in hepatic cysts lined predominantly by stratified squamous epithelium. These lesions appear to have a poor prognosis, although the information in the literature is sparse (32,33).

- Liver metastases

Rarely, certain liver metastases may appear as cystic lesions, usually due to the occurrence of central necrosis. These include metastases from ovarian carcinoma, pancreas, colon, kidney, and neuroendocrine tumors.

6. BILIARY CYSTS

Biliary cysts are cystic dilations that may occur singly or in multiples throughout the biliary tree. Biliary cysts are associated with significant complications, such as ductal strictures, stone formation, cholangitis, rupture, and secondary biliary cirrhosis. In addition, certain types of biliary cysts have a high risk of malignancy. The incidence of biliary cysts has been estimated to be 1:100,000 to 1:150,000, with even wider ranges reported (44). The incidence is higher in some Asian countries (up to 1:1000)). Biliary cysts are more common in women, with a female to male ratio of 3:1 to 4:1. In the past, the majority of cases were reported in children, although more recent series report equal numbers in adults and children.

Classification

The classification scheme defines five types of biliary cyst:

- Type I cysts: account for 50-85 % of all biliary cysts (44). They are characterized by cystic or fusiform dilation of the common bile duct. Type I cysts are further subcategorized (7):
  - Type IA is defined by cystic dilation of the entire extrahepatic biliary tree and is associated with an abnormal pancreaticobiliary junction (APBJ). There is no dilation of the intrahepatic ducts. The cystic duct and gallbladder arise from the dilated common bile duct.
  - Type IB is defined by focal, segmental (often distal) dilation of the extrahepatic bile duct. Type IB cysts are not associated with an APBJ.
  - Type IC is defined by smooth, fusiform (as opposed to cystic) dilation of the entire extrahepatic bile duct. Typically, the dilation extends from the pancreatobiliary junction to the intrahepatic biliary tree. Type IC cysts are associated with an APBJ.
- Type II cysts: account for 2% of biliary cysts. They are true diverticula of the extrahepatic bile duct and communicate with the bile duct through a narrow stalk.
- Type III cysts: account for 1–5% of biliary cysts and are also known as choledochoceles or intraluminal duodenal duplications. Type III cysts are cystic dilations limited to the intraduodenal portion of the distal common bile duct. Choledochoceles can be lined by duodenal or biliary epithelium and may arise embriologically as duodenal duplications involving the ampulla. As many as five subtypes have been described. However, most commonly they are subdivided into:

  - Type IIIA cysts (in which the bile duct and pancreatic duct enter the choledochocele, which then drains into the duodenum at a separate orifice)

- Type IIIB cysts (a diverticulum of the intraduodenal bile duct or common channel) (49).
- Type IV cysts: account for 15 - 35% of cysts. They are defined by the presence of multiple cysts and are subdivided based upon their intrahepatic bile duct involvement. Type IVA cysts have both intrahepatic and extrahepatic cystic dilations, whereas type IVB cysts have multiple extrahepatic cysts but no intrahepatic cysts. Type IVA is the second most common type of biliary cyst and can be differentiated from type IC cysts on the basis of a distinct change in duct caliber at the hilum, or a stricture at the hilum (47).
- Type V cysts: account for 20% of biliary cysts. They are characterized by one or more cystic dilations of the intrahepatic ducts, without extrahepatic duct disease. The presence of multiple saccular or cystic dilations of the intrahepatic ducts is known as Caroli's disease.

Pathogenesis

Several theories of biliary cyst formation have been proposed, and it is likely that no one mechanism accounts for all biliary cysts (46). Cysts may be congenital or acquired (50) and have been associated with a variety of anatomic abnormalities. A genetic or environmental predisposition to biliary cysts is suggested by reports of the familial occurrence of cysts (51) and by the increased incidence in some Asian countries.

Developmental anomalies associated with biliary cysts include:

- Biliary atresia
- Duodenal atresia
- Colonic atresia
- Imperforate anus
- Pancreatic arteriovenous malformation
- Multiseptate gallbladder
- Hemifacial microsomia with extracraniofacial anomalies (OMENS plus syndrome)
- Ventricular septal defect
- Aortic hypoplasia
- Congenital absence of the portal vein
- Heterotopic pancreatic tissue
- Familial adenomatous polyposis
- Autosomal recessive and autosomal dominant polycystic kidney disease

Congenital cysts may result from an unequal proliferation of embryologic biliary epithelial cells before bile duct cannulation is complete. Fetal viral infection may also have a role, as reovirus RNA has been isolated from biliary tissue of neonates with infantile biliary obstruction and biliary cysts (52). In addition, cyst formation may be the result of ductal obstruction or distension during the prenatal or neonatal period.

- Role of an abnormal pancreaticobiliary junction

Acquired cysts may be the result of an abnormal pancreaticobiliary junction (APBJ), also called pancreaticobiliary maljunction. APBJ is a rare congenital anomaly, with a prevalence of 0.03 percent in one population-based series from Japan (53). It is present in about 70% of patients with biliary cysts and may be a significant risk factor for the development of malignancy with the cyst (54). In addition, patients with APBJ without biliary cysts appear to be at a markedly increased risk for gallbladder cancer (55).

APBJ is characterized by a junction of the bile duct and pancreatic duct outside the duodenal wall with a long common duct channel. APBJ may result from failure of the embryological ducts to migrate fully into the duodenum. A long common channel may predispose to reflux of pancreatic juice into the biliary tree since the ductal junction lies outside of the duodenal wall and the sphincter of Oddi (56). This can result in increased amylase levels in bile, intraductal activation of proteolytic enzymes, alterations in bile composition, and theoretically biliary epithelial damage, inflammation, ductal distension, and cyst formation. Elevated sphincter of Oddi pressures have been documented in APBJ(57) and could promote pancreaticobiliary reflux.

Clinical Manifestations

The majority of patients with biliary cysts will present before the age of 10 years (59). Infants with biliary cysts commonly present with conjugated hyperbilirubinemia (80%), failure to thrive, or an abdominal mass (30–60%) (44). The triad of pain, jaundice, and an abdominal mass is found in 11 - 63% of children.

In contrast, chronic and intermittent abdominal pain is the most common presenting symptom (50–96%) in patients older than two (44,60). Intermittent jaundice and recurrent cholangitis are also seen frequently (34 - 55%).

Rarely, biliary cysts present with intraperitoneal rupture, bleeding due to erosion into adjacent vessels or portal hypertension, and secondary biliary cirrhosis due to prolonged biliary obstruction and recurrent cholangitis (59). In addition, type III cysts can case gastric outlet obstruction due to the obstruction of the duodenal lumen or intussusception.

Diagnosis

A biliary cyst should be considered in adults when a dilated portion of the bile duct or ampulla is identified, especially in the absence of biochemical, imaging, or endoscopic evidence of obstruction. Multiple imaging modalities are available, including transabdominal ultrasound, computed tomography, endoscopic retrograde cholangiopancreatography, and magnetic resonance cholangiopancreatography.

A high level of suspicion is required for diagnosis, particularly for type I cysts, which may go undiagnosed unless considered in the differential diagnosis of patients found to have ductal dilation. On the other hand, acute or chronic biliary obstruction may cause marked biliary dilation that mimics a type I cyst.

Such patients usually present with jaundice or elevated serum liver tests, have a readily identifiable obstructing lesion such as a stone, stricture, or mass, and their biliary dilation often improves after appropriate treatment (61). A careful evaluation for an abnormal pancreatobiliary junction may help with diagnosis in indeterminate cases.

Cancer Risk

Biliary cysts are associated with an increased risk of cancer, particularly cholangiocarcinoma (62). The incidence of malignancy varies with age and with the type of cyst.

In a 1983 review of all published series of biliary cysts, the incidence of cancer was 0.7% in patients under 10 years of age, 6.8% in patients 11 to 20 years of age, and 14.3% in patients over 20 years of age (58). In a systematic review from 2007, the incidence of biliary cancer was in the range of 10 – 30% (16% in the largest report), with a mean age at diagnosis of 32 years. However, an incidence of cancer as high as 50% has been reported in older patients.

Most of the cancers occur in type I and type IV cysts. In one series, 68% of the malignancies occurred in patients with type I cysts, and 21% occurred in patients with type IV cysts (63). Patients with type II cysts and type III cysts accounted for 5 and 2% of cases, respectively. Cancer in patients with type III cysts may be limited to those with choledochoceles lined by biliary, rather than duodenal, epithelium (64). Type V cysts (Caroli's disease) have also been associated with a 7 – 15% risk of malignancy (46,62). Multiple studies have described molecular changes that occur during the evolution to malignancy, but their role in diagnosis or management is unclear.

The presence of an abnormal pancreatobiliary junction (APBJ) alone increases the risk of malignancy. In one study, the increased incidence of cholangiocarcinoma in biliary cysts was confined to patients with an APBJ (54). In addition, APBJ appears to increase the risk of biliary and pancreatic malignancy even in patients without a biliary cyst or ductal dilation (52-54).

Nevertheless, evidence clearly points to a 20- to 30-fold increased risk of cholangiocarcinoma in biliary cysts compared with the general population (62). This evidence includes the occurrence of cholangiocarcinoma in patients as young as 10 years of age, the occurrence of synchronous and metachronous biliary cancers, and the subsequent development of cancer in patients with incompletely resected cysts (69).

Management

The approach to management depends upon the type of cyst. In the past, some patients were treated with internal drainage via a cystenterostomy. While effective at treating symptoms, the procedure was associated with significant complications such as ascending cholangitis due to reflux of enteric contents into the cyst and biliary tree, anastomotic stricture formation, and most importantly, a 30% postoperative risk of malignancy (70). Because of these complications, patients requiring treatment now generally undergo cyst excision with hepaticoenterostomy.

Regardless of the type of cyst, patients with ascending cholangitis require treatment with antibiotics and drainage. Drainage can often be obtained via endoscopic retrograde cholangiopancreatography or percutaneous transhepatic cholangiography.

o   Patients with type I, II, and IV cysts usually undergo surgical resection of the cysts due to the significant risk of malignancy, provided they are good surgical candidates.

o   Patients with an abnormal pancreaticobiliary junction and no biliary cyst should consider prophylactic cholecystectomy given their increased risk of gallbladder cancer.

o   Patients with type III cysts (choledochoceles) can often be managed with endoscopic sphincterotomy or endoscopic resection.

o   Intrahepatic cysts may be difficult to resect, and some patients with type V cysts may require liver transplantation.

REFERENCES

[1]   Benhamou, JP, Menu, Y. *Non-parasitic cystic diseases of the liver and intrahepatic biliary tree.* In: Surgery of the liver and biliary tract, 2nd edition, Blumgart, LH (Ed), Churchill Livingstone Inc, New York 1994. p.1197-1200.

[2]   Gadzijev E, Dragan S, Verica FM, et al. *Hepatobiliary cystadenoma protruding into the common bile duct, mimicking complicated hydatid cyst of the liver. Report of a case.* Hepatogastroenterology 1995; 42:1008-10.

[3]   Salemis NS, Georgoulis E, Gourgiotis S, et al. *Spontaneous rupture of a giant non parasitic hepatic cyst presenting as an acute surgical abdomen.* Ann Hepatol 2007; 6:190-3.

[4]   Hanazaki K, Wakabayashi M, Mori H, et al. *Hemorrhage into a simple liver cyst: diagnostic implications of a recent case.* J Gastroenterol 1997; 32:848-51.

[5]   Jones, RS. *Surgical management of non-parasitic liver cysts.* Surgery of the liver and biliary tract, 2nd edition, Blumgart, LH (Ed), Churchill Livingstone, London 1994. p.1211-13.

[6]   Taylor BR, Langer B. *Current surgical management of hepatic cyst disease.* Adv Surg 1997; 31:127-48.

[7]   Burch JC, Jones HE. *Large nonparasitic cyst of the liver simulating an ovarian cyst.* Am J Obstet Gynecol 1952; 63:441-44.

[8]   Dockerty MB, Gray HK, Henson SW Jr. *Benign tumors of the* liver. III. Solitary cysts. Surg Gynecol Obstet 1956; 103:607-12.

[9]   Nisenbaum HL, Rowling SE. *Ultrasound of focal hepatic lesions.* Semin Roentgenol 1995; 30:324-46.

[10] Hagiwara A, Inoue Y, Shutoh T, et al. *Haemorrhagic hepatic cyst: a differential diagnosis of cystic tumour.* Br J Radiol 2001; 74:270-72.

[11] Regev A, Reddy KR, Berho M, et al. *Large cystic lesions of the liver in adults: a 15-year experience in a tertiary center.* J Am Coll Surg 2001; 193:36-45.

[12] Gigot JF, Legrand M, Hubens G, et al. *Laparoscopic treatment of nonparasitic liver cysts: adequate selection of patients and surgical technique.* World J Surg 1996; 20:556-61.

[13] Blonski WC, Campbell MS, Faust T, et al. *Successful aspiration and ethanol sclerosis of a large, symptomatic, simple liver cyst: case presentation and review of the literature.* World J Gastroenterol 2006; 12:2949-54.

[14] Wittig JH, Burns R, Longmire WP Jr. *Jaundice associated with polycystic liver disease.* Am J Surg 1978; 136:383-6.

[15] Zacherl J, Scheuba C, Imhof M, et al. *Long-term results after laparoscopic unroofing of solitary symptomatic congenital liver cysts.* Surg Endosc 2000; 14:59-62.

[16] Garcea G, Pattenden CJ, Stephenson J, et al. *Nine-year single-center experience with nonparastic liver cysts: diagnosis and management.* Dig Dis Sci 2007; 52:185-91.

[17] Koperna T, Vogl S, Satzinger U, et al. *Nonparasitic cysts of the liver: results and options of surgical treatment.* World J Surg 1997; 21:850-4.

[18] Larssen TB, Viste A, Jensen DK, et al. *Single-session alcohol sclerotherapy in benign symptomatic hepatic cysts.* Acta Radiol 1997; 38:993-7.

[19] Okano A, Hajiro K, Takakuwa H, et al. *Alcohol sclerotherapy of hepatic cysts: its effect in relation to ethanol concentration.* Hepatol Res 2000; 17:179-184.

[20] Wernet A, Sibert A, Paugam-Burtz C, et al. *Ethanol-induced coma after therapeutic ethanol injection of a hepatic cyst.* Anesthesiology 2008; 108:328-9.

[21] Mazza OM, Fernandez DL, Pekolj J, et al. *Management of nonparasitic hepatic cysts.* J Am Coll Surg 2009; 209:733-9.

[22] Gamblin TC, Holloway SE, Heckman JT, et al. *Laparoscopic resection of benign hepatic cysts: a new standard.* J Am Coll Surg 2008; 207:731-6.

[23] Loehe F, Globke B, Marnoto R, et al. *Long-term results after surgical treatment of nonparasitic hepatic cysts.* Am J Surg 2010; 200:23-31.

[24] Ishak KG, Willis GW, Cummins SD, et al. *Biliary cystadenoma and cystadenocarcinoma: report of 14 cases and review of the literature.* Cancer 1977; 39:322-38.

[25] Wheeler DA, Edmondson HA. *Cystadenoma with mesenchymal stroma (CMS) in the liver and bile ducts. A clinicopathologic study of 17 cases, 4 with malignant change.* Cancer 1985; 56:1434-45.

[26] Devaney K, Goodman ZD, Ishak KG. *Hepatobiliary cystadenoma and cystadenocarcinoma. A light microscopic and immunohistochemical study of 70 patients.* Am J Surg Pathol 1994; 18:1078-91.

[27] Di Bisceglie AM. *Malignant neoplasms of the liver.* In: Chiff's Diseases of the Liver, 8th edition, Schiff, ER, Sorrell, MF, Maddrey, WC (Eds), Lippincott-Raven, Philadephia 1999. p.1281-87.

[28] Hai S, Hirohashi K, Uenishi T, et al. *Surgical management of cystic hepatic neoplasms.* J Gastroenterol 2003; 38:759-64.

[29] Tomimatsu M, Okuda H, Saito A, et al. *A case of biliary cystadenocarcinoma with morphologic and histochemical features of hepatocytes.* Cancer 1989; 64:1323-8.

[30] Iemoto Y, Kondo Y, Fukamachi S. *Biliary cystadenocarcinoma with peritoneal carcinomatosis.* Cancer 1981; 48:1664-7.

[31] Devine P, Ucci AA. *Biliary cystadenocarcinoma arising in a congenital cyst.* Hum Pathol 1985; 16:92-94.

[32] Vick DJ, Goodman ZD, Deavers MT, et al. *Ciliated hepatic foregut cyst: a study of six cases and review of the literature.* Am J Surg Pathol 1999; 23:671-7.

[33] Hsieh CB, Chen CJ, Yu JC, et al. *Primary squamous cell carcinoma of the liver arising from a complex liver cyst: report of a case.* Surg Today 2005; 35:328.

[34] Dervenis C, Delis S, Avgerinos C, et al. *Changing concepts in the management of liver hydatid disease.* J Gastrointest Surg 2005; 9:869-77.

[35] Brunetti E, Kern P, Vuitton DA. *Writing Panel for the WHO-IWGE. Expert consensus for the diagnosis and treatment of cystic and alveolar echinococcosis in humans.* Acta Trop 2010; 114:1-19.

[36] Guidelines for treatment of cystic and alveolar echinococcosis in humans. *WHO Informal Working Group on Echinococcosis.* Bull World Health Organ 1996; 74:231-42.

[37] Safioleas MC, Misiakos EP, Kouvaraki M, et al. *Hydatid disease of the liver: a continuing surgical problem.* Arch Surg 2006; 141:1101-8.

[38] Junghanss T, da Silva AM, Horton J, et al. *Clinical management of cystic echinococcosis: state of the art, problems, and perspectives.* Am J Trop Med Hyg 2008; 79:301-11.

[39] Arif SH, Wani NA, Zargar SA, et al. *Albendazole as an adjuvant to the standard surgical management of hydatid cyst liver.* Int J Surg 2008; 6:448-51.

[40] Nasseri Moghaddam S, Abrishami A, Malekzadeh R. *Percutaneous needle aspiration, injection, and reaspiration with or without benzimidazole coverage for uncomplicated hepatic hydatid cysts.* Cochrane Database Syst Rev 2006; CD003623.

[41] Smego RA Jr, Bhatti S, Khaliq AA, et al. *Percutaneous aspiration-injection-reaspiration drainage plus albendazole or mebendazole for hepatic cystic echinococcosis: a meta-analysis.* Clin Infect Dis 2003; 37:1073-83.

[42] World Health Organization (WHO) *Informal Working Group of Echinococcosis. Puncture, Aspiration, Injection, Re-Aspiration. An option for the treatment of cystic echinococcosis, p. 1–40.* Document WHO/CDS/CSR/SPH/2001.6. Geneva, Switzerland: WHO; 2001. pp. 1–40.

[43] Ruiz-Tovar J, Lopez-Buenadicha A, Páramo J, et al. *Massive recurrence of cyst hydatid disease in the proximal thigh: unsuccessful conservative treatment with percutaneous aspiration, ethanol injection, and reaspiration.* Am Surg 2009;75:439-441.

[44] Lipsett PA, Pitt HA, Colombani PM, et al. *Choledochal cyst disease. A changing pattern of presentation.* Ann Surg 1994; 220:644-52.

[45] O'Neill JA Jr. *Choledochal cyst.* Curr Probl Surg 1992; 29:361-410.

[46] Singham J, Yoshida EM, Scudamore CH. *Choledochal cysts: part 1 of 3: classification and pathogenesis.* Can J Surg 2009; 52:434-40.

[47] Todani T, Watanabe Y, Toki A, et al. *Classification of congenital biliary cystic disease: special reference to type Ic and IVA cysts with primary ductal stricture.* J Hepatobiliary Pancreat Surg 2003; 10:340-4.

[48] Cha SW, Park MS, Kim KW, et al. *Choledochal cyst and anomalous pancreaticobiliary ductal union in adults: radiological spectrum and complications.* J Comput Assist Tomogr 2008; 32:17-22.

[49] Sarris GE, Tsang D. *Choledochocele: case report, literature review, and a proposed classification.* Surgery 1989; 105:408-14.

[50] Han SJ, Hwang EH, Chung KS, et al. *Acquired choledochal cyst from anomalous pancreatobiliary duct union.* J Pediatr Surg 1997; 32:1735-8.

[51] Iwata F, Uchida A, Miyaki T, et al. *Familial occurrence of congenital bile duct cysts.* J Gastroenterol Hepatol 1998; 13:316-9.

[52] Tyler KL, Sokol RJ, Oberhaus SM, et al. *Detection of reovirus RNA in hepatobiliary tissues from patients with extrahepatic biliary atresia and choledochal cysts.* Hepatology 1998; 27:1475-82.

[53] Yamao K, Mizutani S, Nakazawa S, et al. *Prospective study of the detection of anomalous connections of pancreatobiliary ducts during routine medical examinations.* Hepatogastroenterology 1996; 43:1238-45.

[54] Song HK, Kim MH, Myung SJ, et al. *Choledochal cyst associated the with anomalous union of pancreaticobiliary duct (AUPBD) has a more grave clinical course than choledochal cyst alone.* Korean J Intern Med 1999; 14:1-8.

[55] Funabiki T, Matsubara T, Miyakawa S, et al. *Pancreaticobiliary maljunction and carcinogenesis to biliary and pancreatic malignancy.* Langenbecks Arch Surg 2009; 394:159-69.

[56] Matsumoto S, Tanaka M, Ikeda S, et al. *Sphincter of Oddi motor activity in patients with anomalous pancreaticobiliary junction.* Am J Gastroenterol 1991; 86:831-4.

[57] Craig AG, Chen LD, Saccone GT, et al. *Sphincter of Oddi dysfunction associated with choledochal cyst.* J Gastroenterol Hepatol 2001; 16:230-4.

[58] Voyles CR, Smadja C, Shands WC, et al. *Carcinoma in choledochal cysts. Age-related incidence.* Arch Surg 1983; 118:986-8.

[59] Singham J, Yoshida EM, Scudamore CH. *Choledochal cysts: part 2 of 3: Diagnosis.* Can J Surg 2009; 52:506-11.

[60] Singham J, Schaeffer D, Yoshida E, et al. *Choledochal cysts: analysis of disease pattern and optimal treatment in adult and paediatric patients.* HPB (Oxford) 2007; 9:383-7.

[61] Aggarwal S, Kumar A, Roy S, et al. *Massive dilatation of the common bile duct resembling a choledochal cyst.* Trop Gastroenterol 2001; 22:219-20.

[62] Søreide K, Søreide JA. *Bile duct cyst as precursor to biliary tract cancer.* Ann Surg Oncol 2007; 14:1200-11.

[63] Todani T, Tabuchi K, Watanabe Y, et al. *Carcinoma arising in the wall of congenital bile duct cysts.* Cancer 1979; 44:1134-41.

[64] Ohtsuka T, Inoue K, Ohuchida J, et al. *Carcinoma arising in choledochocele.* Endoscopy 2001; 33:614-9.

[65] Elnemr A, Ohta T, Kayahara M, et al. *Anomalous pancreaticobiliary ductal junction without bile duct dilatation in gallbladder cancer.* Hepatogastroenterology 2001; 48:382-6.

[66] Sugiyama M, Abe N, Tokuhara M, et al. *Pancreatic carcinoma associated with anomalous pancreaticobiliary junction.* Hepatogastroenterology 2001; 48:1767-9.

[67] Sugiyama M, Atomi Y. *Anomalous pancreaticobiliary junction without congenital choledochal cyst.* Br J Surg 1998; 85:911-6.

[68] Kobayashi S, Asano T, Yamasaki M, et al. *Risk of bile duct carcinogenesis after excision of extrahepatic bile ducts in pancreaticobiliary maljunction.* Surgery 1999; 126:939-44.

[69] Watanabe Y, Toki A, Todani T. *Bile duct cancer developed after cyst excision for choledochal cyst.* J Hepatobiliary Pancreat Surg 1999; 6:207-12.

[70] Tao KS, Lu YG, Wang T, et al. *Procedures for congenital choledochal cysts and curative effect analysis in adults.* Hepatobiliary Pancreat Dis Int 2002; 1:442-5.

[71] Morar R, Feldman C. *Pulmonary echinococcosis.* Eur Respir J 2003; 21:1069-77.

[72] Dhar P, Chaudhary A, Desai R, et al. *Current trends in the diagnosis and management of cystic hydatid disease of the liver.* J Commun Dis 1996; 28:221-30.

[73] Safioleas M, Misiakos E, Manti C, et al. *Diagnostic evaluation and surgical management of hydatid disease of the liver.* World J Surg 1994; 18:859-65.

[74] Salama H, Farid Abdel-Wahab M, Strickland GT. *Diagnosis and treatment of hepatic hydatid cysts with the aid of echo-guided percutaneous cyst puncture.* Clin Infect Dis 1995; 21:1372-6.

[75] Suwan Z. *Sonographic findings in hydatid disease of the liver: comparison with other imaging methods.* Ann Trop Med Parasitol 1995; 89:261-9.

[76] Bhatia G. *Echinococcus.* Semin Respir Infect 1997; 12:171-86.

[77] McManus DP, Zhang W, Li J. *Echinococcosis.* Lancet 2003; 362:1295-304.

[78] Kervancioglu R, Bayram M, Elbeyli L. *CT findings in pulmonary hydatid disease.* Acta Radiol 1999; 40:510-4.

[79] el-Tahir MI, Omojola MF, Malatani T, et al. *Hydatid disease of the liver: evaluation of ultrasound and computed tomography.* Br J Radiol 1992; 65:390-2.

[80] Tüzün M, Altinörs N, Arda IS,et al. *Cerebral hydatid disease CT and MR findings.* Clin Imaging 2002; 26:353-7.81.

[81] Siles-Lucas MM, Gottstein BB. *Molecular tools for the diagnosis of cystic and alveolar echinococcosis.* Trop Med Int Health 2001; 6:463-75.

[82] Khuroo MS, Dar MY, Yattoo GN, et al. Percutaneous drainage versus albendazole therapy in hepatic hydatidosis: a prospective, randomized study. Gastroenterology 1993; 104:1452-9.

In: Cysts: Causes, Diagnosis and Treatment Options
Editors: A. Mendes Ortiz and A. Jimenez Moreno

ISBN: 978-1-62081-315-7
© 2012 Nova Science Publishers, Inc.

Chapter 5

NON-PARASITIC BENIGN LIVER CYSTS

J. M. Ramia*, R. De la Plaza, J. Quiñones and J. Garcia-Parreño

Hepato-Pancreato-Biliary Surgical Service
Department of Surgery, Hospital Universitario de Guadalajara
Guadalajara, Spain

ABSTRACT

Liver cysts are a heterogeneous group of diseases with different aetiology and incidence. Frequently, they are asymptomatic but symptomatic cases cause similar clinical signs and symptoms. The diagnosis of these cysts is now more frequent due to the increasing number or abdominal radiological explorations (abdominal ultrasound or CT) performed for other medical reasons. They are classified as congenital, traumatic, parasitic, or neoplastic cysts. The congenital cystic tumours are the most frequent type including simple liver cyst and polycystic hepatic disease. Other less common lesions are: hepatic cystadenoma, ciliated embryonic cyst, Caroli Disease and a miscellaneous group. Liver hydatidosis is the most frequent parasitic liver cyst in many countries. We perform in this chapter a review of non-parasitic liver cyst focusing in most adequate treatment that includes from clinical follow-up to liver transplantation. The possibility of performing some surgical procedures by laparoscopy approach has opened some controversies in the management of liver cysts that are not well answered in medical literature.

NON-PARASITIC BENIGN LIVER CYSTS

Hepatic cysts (HC) are a heterogeneous group of diseases with a different aetiology and prevalence, but are clinically similar.[1–4] They can be classified as congenital, traumatic, parasitic and neoplastic. [5–10] The congenital type is the most important one and includes

* Correspondence: J.M. Ramia, C/General Moscardó 26, 5-1, Madrid, 28020,. Spain. E-mail: jose_ramia@hotmail.com; Telephone: 0034-616292056.

simple cyst (SC) and polycystic liver disease (PLD). [8, 9, 11–13] HC are diagnosed incidentally, as they are usually asymptomatic, benign and more frequent in women. [2–4, 6, 14–17] Their incidence is unknown but it is estimated that 5% of the population have non-parasitic HC. [7, 8, 15, 17–22]

Simple Cyst

The SC is the most common liver injury, with a prevalence in the adult population of between 0.1% and 7%. [5, 6, 9–12, 20, 22–31] It is filled with serous fluid and has no communication with the biliary tree. [10, 12, 16, 23, 24] It is more common in women, with a ratio of 2:1 for asymptomatic and 9:1 for symptomatic SC. [2, 5, 8, 17, 19, 22, 24, 27, 29, 31]. It is probably due to an aberrant bile duct losing communication with the biliary tree, [1, 5, 8, 10, 12, 14, 18, 22, 24, 27–30, 32] and cases of spontaneous disappearance have been reported. [30]

Macroscopically, it has a spherical or ovoid shape, unilocular and without septa. Its size ranges from a few millimeters to more than 20 cm, and 60% of patients have a single lesion. [6, 23, 24] Unlike PLD, multiple SC occupy less than 50% of a patient's liver. [6, 17] Microscopically, the SC has a column monolayer epithelium, similar to the biliary one, that may become necrotic if the intracystic pressure is high. [5, 6, 23, 24, 27, 29, 30] There is no surrounding stroma in small SC and only a thin layer of connective tissue in large ones. [6, 24]

SC is usually asymptomatic and diagnosed incidentally. [9–12, 17, 22–25, 28, 29, 31–33] When symptomatic (10%– 15%), the most common symptom is abdominal pain. [5, 14, 17, 18, 22, 24, 27, 28, 30, 32] Other symptoms include nausea and vomiting, postprandial fullness, shoulder pain, dyspnea and palpable abdominal tumor, etc. [5, 11, 12, 16–18, 20, 22, 24, 28, 31, 32] Analytical studies provide normal results unless there is compression of the biliary tree. Some SC present with high levels of intracystic CA19-9. [9, 18, 34] SC complications occur in 5% of patients. [11, 20, 23] The two most common complications are infection (Figure 1), often monomicrobial by E. coli, and bleeding. [2, 11, 16, 20, 23, 26, 32] Other less common ones are as follows: traumatic or spontaneous rupture, torsion, compression of surrounding structures such as the inferior vena cava; portal vein, causing portal hypertension; the bile duct, producing cholestasis, cholangitis and jaundice; fistulisation to the duodenum or biliary tree; and exceptionally, malignisation. [2, 7–9, 11, 16, 20, 22–24, 26,28, 31, 32, 35– 41]

Intracystic haemorrhage usually occurs in elderly patients with large SC. [13, 33] The most common symptoms are rapid growth and abdominal pain. [2, 12, 31, 33] If bleeding is significant, it may lead to compressive thrombosis of the inferior vena cava. [13, 20, 36] The intracystic haematic content may mimic a hepatic cystadenoma (HCy). [13, 33, 38] Contrast ultrasound and magnetic resonance imaging (MRI) are useful for the diagnosis of intracystic haemorrhage. [2, 12, 42] A bleeding SC must be treated surgically to prevent future complications, [13, 23] although percutaneous drainage, embolization and observation, if it is not infected, have been used in patients with severe comorbidities. [13]

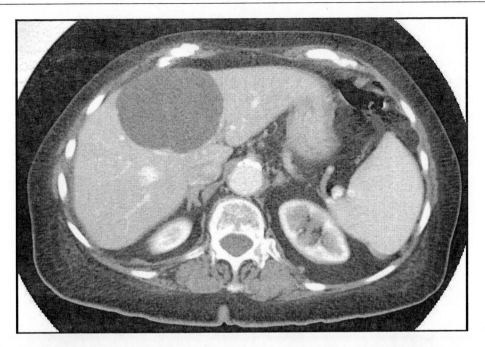

Figure 1. CT: Infected simple liver cyst.

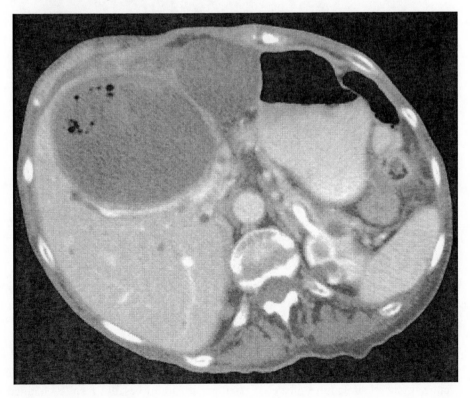

Figure 2. CT: simple liver cyst.

The most cost-effective imaging method for SC is abdominal ultrasound. The radiographic features are typical: a circular or oval anechoic lesion, non-septated, with posterior enhancement caused by dense echoes behind the SC due to intracystic fluid. [5, 11, 23, 24, 42] A CT scan confirms the presence of avascular cystic lesions with water density without contrast enhancement (Figure 2). [11] MRI is useful for the diagnosis and detection of intracystic complications: the SC is observed as a T2 homogeneous hyperintense lesion without contrast enhancement and low intensity on T1. [9, 11, 23] Differential diagnosis arises with the hydatid cyst, especially in endemic areas, HCy and cystic metastases. [1, 10, 14, 18, 24, 43]

Treatment is needed only if there are complications, and periodic monitoring suffices for asymptomatic patients. [1, 5, 12, 14, 15, 17, 22, 24, 25, 27–29, 31, 43] The size of the cyst itself is not an indication for surgery, although large ones are usually symptomatic. [2, 3, 14, 18, 31] Treatment options may be non-surgical (puncture aspiration with or without injection of sclerosing agents) or surgical, [14, 22, 28–30, 32, 44] which are divided into conservative procedures: fenestration, and other techniques now practically abandoned (cystojejunostomy or marsupialisation); or radical (cystectomy or hepatic resection). [3, 12, 17, 25, 26, 29, 32, 44]

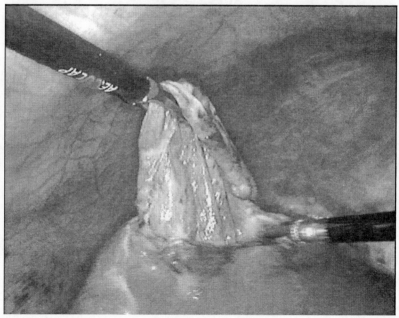

Figure 3. Laparoscopic fenestration of liver cyst.

Aspiration under ultrasound/CT control may relieve the symptoms, but relapse is the norm. It makes sense to apply it only for patients at high surgical risk, as a diagnostic technique, in infected cysts or to find out whether the cyst causes the symptoms. [1–3, 5, 6, 11, 12, 15, 17, 18, 22, 23, 28, 29, 32] The instillation of sclerosing agents (e.g., alcohol, minocycline, monoethanolamine oleate or pantopaque) improves the results obtained with aspiration but has a high recurrence rate (20%–90%) and complications: pain during the procedure, alcohol poisoning, cholangitis or eosinophilia. [2, 9, 11, 12, 14, 16, 18, 22, 28, 29, 31] The presence of a coagulation disorder, intracystic bleeding or SC communication with the biliary tree contraindicates the use of puncturing. [1, 11, 12, 14, 16, 29]

Fenestration is a technique that can be performed by laparotomy or laparoscopy. [12, 22, 26, 28, 32, 45, 46] Its surgical risk is low, but long-term results are short-lived since late relapse is common. Laparoscopic fenestration was first described by Z'graggen in 1991 and has become the most commonly performed procedure in solitary symptomatic SC. [3, 6, 17, 18, 22, 27– 29, 43, 47, 48]

Laparoscopic fenestration (LF) starts with the puncture of the cyst for an analytical study (tumour markers, amylase, bilirubin and LDH), as well as a microbiological and cytological study of the intracystic fluid. The visible part of the SC is then dried with a hook, dissecting sealer, cutting stapler and is extracted into a sample bag for later histological analysis (Figure 3). [2, 5, 27, 28, 31, 32] If there are multiple connected cysts, fenestration of the deep cysts can be performed via the external cysts. [11, 45] The windows made must be large enough to ensure permeability of the communication and prevent the SC from filling. [6, 11, 15, 28] A biopsy must be performed on any suspicious intracystic node. [12, 31] Fulguration of the unresected cystic epithelium has been performed with argon, electro-cautery, and other similar tools. [12, 14, 25, 26, 28, 29, 31, 49] Currently, laparotomic fenestration is rarely indicated. [31]

The percentage of complications after LF of SC is between 0% and 18%. [5, 12, 17, 18, 31] These include the following: abdominal hydatid cyst spread if there is an incorrect diagnosis, post-fenestration ascites, air embolism, pleural effusion, dyspnoea, biloma and haemorrhage. [12, 29, 43, 47] The rate of recurrence of symptoms is between 4% and 44%. [5, 14, 15, 17, 18, 26, 28, 29, 31, 43, 48] Factors favouring recurrence after LF are: cysts centrally located or on the posterior right part, limited resection of the visible cyst wall, previously operated cysts, and the use of a hook instead of a dissecting sealer for resection. [14, 15, 18, 25, 28] The very frequent radiological recurrence after LF is not always accompanied by the appearance of symptoms. [17]

Total cystectomy and hepatic resection are techniques performed occasionally. [2, 5, 11, 12, 14, 15, 22, 29, 31, 44] There is a publication on radiofrequency treatment of SC. [50]

The treatment for patients with infected SC is percutaneous puncture and antibiotics to improve the symptoms and provide a reliable diagnosis, deciding the most appropriate treatment later. [7]

Polycystic Liver Disease

Polycystic liver disease (PLD) has a prevalence of between 0.05% and 0.6%. It consists of multiple hepatic cysts occupying more than 50% of the liver parenchyma. It is as an inherited autosomal dominant disease, and usually occurs in combination with polycystic kidney disease or cysts in other organs (pancreas, spleen, ovaries and lung, although rarely in the latter). [1, 2, 6, 11, 31, 34, 45, 46, 51–64] One-third of patients with PLD never develop kidney cysts, and these patients have genetic alterations on chromosome 19p13.2- 13.1 (PRKSCH) and 6q (SEC63). This is different to patients with hepatorenal polycystic disease, with alterations on chromosomes 4 and 16 (PKD1 and 2). [52, 55, 60, 61, 65–72] Patients with only PLD have larger cysts but with fewer complications than patients with hepatorenal polycystic disease. [52, 66]

PLD is more common in women, who also tend to have more and larger cysts. [46, 60, 64, 66, 73] Patients with PLD also have a higher incidence of intracranial aneurysms. [11, 31,

51, 62, 64, 71, 72] Liver injury in PLD can be microcystic, macrocystic or biliary hamartomas (von Meyenburg complexes) distributed evenly over the liver and peribiliary areas. [52, 58, 61, 69] The normal parenchyma shows fibrosis and vascular changes. [63] Cysts usually contain clear fluid and histologically are lined by cuboidal epithelium. [58, 61, 69] The cysts grow in size, number and volume with age. [65]

PLD cysts are usually asymptomatic. [45, 51, 52, 57, 58, 60, 61, 72] When symptoms occur, due to increased volume or compression of adjacent structures, they are similar to those of SC. [31, 46, 52, 54, 55, 58, 60–65, 67, 72, 74, 75] Complications are more common in symptomatic patients: for example, cyst infection, rupture, torsion, intracystic bleeding, portal hypertension causing ascites and/or oesophageal varices, compression of the vena cava, biliary obstruction or cystocutaneous fistula. [45, 51, 52, 55, 57, 58, 60, 61, 65, 67, 68, 72, 76] Cystic infection or rupture is more common in patients with a kidney transplant, possibly due to immunosuppression. Most symptomatic patients(75%) have palpable hepatomegaly. [54, 61, 62]Stigmata of liver disease and acute liver failure are rare. [60, 77] Diagnosis of PLD can be made by ultrasound, helical CT and MRI. [55, 58, 60, 61, 67, 72] CT is better at defining the extent of the liver disease and the involvement of adjacent organs. [31] It shows multiple hypoattenuating liver lesions of various sizes with well-defined margins and no contrast enhancement (Figure 4). [60, 72] In MRI, the lesions are of low intensity on T1 and hyperintense on T2, 61 and this is very useful for determining intracystic bleeding. [63] The liver biochemical profile is usually normal or slightly altered. [2, 52, 55, 60, 61, 64, 72] The serum CA19-9 may be increased, and the intracystic one is usually very high, especially in large cysts. [59]

Patients with asymptomatic PLD require no treatment. [2, 52, 53, 55, 57, 58, 62, 74] There is no consensus on how to treat symptomatic patients. [2, 27, 31, 45, 53, 55, 57, 60, 61, 63, 65, 72] The goal of treatment is to reduce the size of the cysts, without compromising liver function, and achieve the longest possible period without symptoms. [51]

The choice of treatment must be based on the size and extent of the cysts and the presence or not of complications. Gigot devised a classification that defines a therapeutic strategy and divides the cysts into the following: Type 1, a few large cysts between 7 and 10 cm; Type 2, multiple medium- sized cysts (5–7 cm); and Type 3, multiple medium and small cysts (less than 5 cm). [26, 31, 51, 72, 78] Li and Schnelldorf proposed new classifications which have not been used as much. [51, 74]

Type 1 patients can opt for LF of the accessible dominant cyst(s) or puncture. [1] LF results in a reduction of 12.5% in cystic volume (range: 9.4%–24.7%) which produces a clinical improvement (less bloating and postprandial fullness), and a recurrence of 4.5%–16%. [1, 14, 25, 26, 45, 60, 61, 67, 74, 78] In some cases (e.g., infected cyst or high surgical risk), a percutaneous puncture can be performed to temporarily improve the symptoms. [1, 2, 26, 61, 78] Its advantage is minimum morbidity and mortality, but the disadvantages are the high recurrence rate and low reduction in mass. [46, 53, 58, 61, 67, 72, 79] There are 2 procedures for Type 2 patients: fenestration and liver resection, or a combination of both. Both have significant morbidity, and long-term palliation of the symptoms is not achieved. [3, 7, 15]

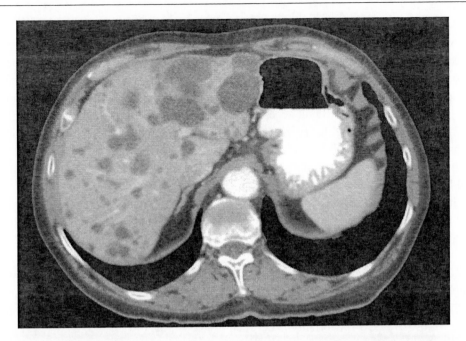

Figure 4. CT: Polycystic liver disease.

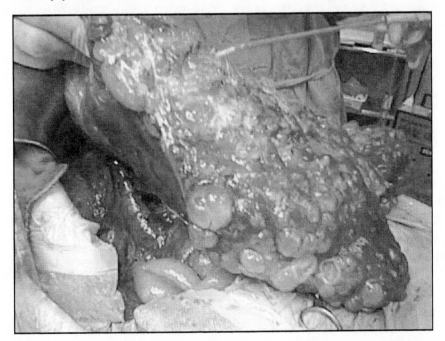

Figure 5. Liver transplantation in Polycystic Liver Disease made in Hospital La Fe, Valencia (Spain).

Fenestration was classically performed by laparotomy by draining the internal cysts into the most superficial ones. [45, 51, 61, 72] Fenestration does not achieve the results expected due to the growth of other small or inaccessible cysts, and for not managing to collapse the liver easily due to its rigidity. [11, 31, 45, 46, 61] In recent years there have been small series of LF in patients with PLD. [26, 31, 45, 60, 67, 78] Comparing both approaches, laparotomic fenestration results in a reduction in volume of 43%, a mean recurrence rate of 17% (11%–

26%), a morbidity between 0% and 56% and a mortality between 0% and 11%. [6, 25, 26, 72] LF obtains an initial improvement in symptoms for over 70% of patients, recurrence is between 0% and 54%, [26, 31, 45, 60, 61] mortality is practically nil and morbidity between 0% and 67% (including ascites, bleeding, biliary fistula and pleural effusion). [26, 45, 48, 67, 72] The technical problems of LF are mistaking a cyst for a large venous trunk, leading to cataclysmic bleeding; and difficult access to the intrahepatic cysts or posterior segments. [25, 45, 51, 53, 61, 75] The published results do not give a clear preference for laparotomy or laparoscopic fenestration. [51]

Hepatic resection is occasionally used, but is the method of choice when the patient has portal hypertension and/or cysts situated in an anatomical region of the liver.

The combination of resection and fenestration of peripheral cysts and communication with the innermost ones is the technique with the best results, with a reduction in volume of 75% and a recurrence rate of 15%. [1, 26, 46, 51, 53, 62, 63, 67, 69] The advantages are: reduction in volume, complex cyst elimination, and regeneration of healthy liver parts. [63] Morbidity ranges between 20% and 100%, including vascular lesions, biliary lesions, postoperative ascites, which is very difficult to resolve as it exceeds the peritoneal absorption capacity (900 ml/day), insufficient postoperative liver volume and kinking of the liver. [45, 46, 51, 61–63, 67, 72, 74] Mortality is between 0% and 11%. [46, 51, 53, 63, 67, 72, 74] The main disadvantages of this technique are high morbidity and mortality; it is not applicable to patients with a severe preoperative hepatorenal situation and, when it fails, there is little choice for the patient other than a liver transplant. It is always recommended to perform a cholecystectomy with cholangiography to prevent biliary leakage. [58, 63] Fenestration of the cysts near the hepatic veins and vena cava is important to prevent future compression complications. [63, 74]

Type 3 can be treated by a combination of fenestration and/or resection or liver transplant (Figure 5). [1, 26, 63, 74] If the PLD-affected areas are close and leave enough viable parenchyma, resection with fenestration is feasible. However, when it is very diffuse, or the remaining volume is less than 30%, or there are histological changes in the liver parenchyma or there is renal failure, a transplant is indicated before any complica-tions appear. [31, 63, 64, 68, 78] In 1988, Kwok performed the first PLD-induced liver transplant. Since then there have been 600 cases in Europe and PLD consists of 0.5% of indications for liver transplantation. [51, 56, 64, 68, 73, 77, 80, 81] The most common indication is the lethal exhaustion syndrome (cachexia, fatigue and pain). [72] Women comprise 90% of transplant recipients, hepatorenal affectation is 90%, but only 53% are kidney transplants. [56, 63, 64, 68, 73, 74, 77, 80–83] Morbidity is 85% and perioperative mortality is 12.5%, due mainly to the poor pre-operative condition. Survival at 5 years is 85%. [56, 63, 64, 67, 73, 74, 77, 80–83] Palliation of the symptoms is excellent. [56, 63, 64, 67, 73, 74, 77, 80–83]

These transplants are often complex due to previous surgery and the large size of the liver. [63, 67, 77] Traditionally, it was recommended to start surgery via the hepatic hilum, use the veno-venous bypass and the classical technique with resection of the inferior vena cava, [65] but the piggyback option is feasible in a large percentage of patients. [63, 81]

There are several arguments against performing a liver transplant in PLD: it is a benign disease, there is usually hepatocellular failure, indefinite immunosuppressive therapy, surgery with associated morbidity and mortality and lack of donations. [1, 63, 64, 77, 81] The arguments in favour are: good results and improved quality of life after transplantation. [61,

64, 67] The right time to perform liver transplantation and the conve-nience of a hepatorenal transplant is a complex decision. [63, 64, 67, 77]

Other therapeutic measures include treatment with octreotide and analogues but these have not been successful. [34, 74] A multicentre study of lanreotide obtained a reduction in cystic volume of 2.9%. [65] Placing a stent in the vena cava in patients with intractable ascites caused by hepatomegaly may be effective. [54]

Hepatobiliary Cystadenomas

Hepatobiliary cystadenomas (HCy) are rare liver tumours, [6, 84–93] comprising 5% of total hepatic cysts. [4, 84, 85, 87–97] Middle-aged women account for 85% of them. [3, 4, 84–87, 89–94, 96, 97] Its histogenesis is unknown. [90, 92–94, 97] In 1985, 2 subtypes of HCy were defined, according to the presence or not of ovarian-like mesenchymal stroma. [4, 87, 88, 90, 91, 98] The HCy without stroma are more common in men, and become malignant more often. [87, 94, 96, 99] There is a sub-type of HCy without stroma with acidophilic cells that only occurs in men and is considered a semi-malignant variant. [91] It is not known if the malignant variant (cystadenocarcinoma) is an evolution from a HCy or an initially malignant tumour. [87, 90, 91] The rate of malignancy may reach 30%. [84]

HCy are multiloculated, well-defined, solitary lesions, usually with internal septations, papillary projections or nodules on the wall of the HCy or septa. At the microscopic level, they have the following layers: simple cuboidal or columnar monolayer epithelium, mesenchymal stroma (absent in the variant without stroma) and an outer layer of dense connective tissue. [4, 6, 84, 86, 87, 90–94, 96–98, 100, 10]1 The intracys- tic fluid may be cloudy or clear with a gelatinous or mucinous appearance. [87, 94] HCy is variable in size (1.5–30 cm). [85, 87, 88, 93, 95] There may occasionally be communication between the HCy and the biliary tree. It is associated with mucinous cystic tumours of the pancreas. [86, 90, 96]

Most HCy are asymptomatic and are found incidentally. [85, 87, 90–94] The symptoms it causes are similar to those of SC. [4, 21, 85–91, 93, 94, 97, 100] Possible complications include intracystic haemorrhage, compression or obstruction of the bile duct, ascites, bacterial overinfection, rupture, recurrence and malignisation. [85, 89–91, 94, 97]

Analytical studies are usually normal, with elevated liver function results if there is compression of the biliary tree. [21, 93, 94, 96] Markers in the intracystic fluid are high, especially for CA19-9. [84, 93, 94, 102] The presence of CA19-9 in the epithelium of HCy has been demonstrated immunohistochemically. [4, 13, 86–88, 91, 92, 97, 102, 103]The ultrasound image shows an ovoid anechoic cystic mass with multiple hyperechoic internal septa and papillary projections in the septa or cyst wall. [4, 86, 87, 91, 92] The CT image shows a multilobulated, well-defined, thick-walled cystic mass of low density, and usually has internal septa, mural nodules, and/or papillary projections with contrast enhancement. [4, 6, 87, 91, 92, 97] MRI is useful for evaluating the intracystic content features. [94] Puncturing is not recommended due to the low diagnostic sensitivity and risk of spread. [4, 13, 91] Correct preoperative diagnosis is between 30% and 95%. [84] The presence of a significant solid component (nodular solid masses or marked parietal thickening), intracystic haemorrhage, wall calcifications, and the combination of nodules and septa are suggestive of malignancy. [87, 91, 95–97]

HCy treatment is complete surgical resection, as it is a potentially malignant lesion, which commonly relapses after partial surgery due to the inability to preoperatively distinguish between HCy and cystadenocarcinoma. [3, 4, 6, 10, 21, 84–86, 88–90, 94, 96, 97, 99, 100] The decision to perform complete enucleation or anatomic resection depends on the location of the HCy. [4, 89, 91, 92, 94, 99] HCy with mesenchymal stroma is more easily enucleated. [91]

Patients diagnosed preoperatively for SC who undergo a LF with a final diagnosis of HCy must be operated on for complete excision. [91, 93]

Ciliated Hepatic Foregut Cyst

Ciliated hepatic foregut cyst (CHFC) is an uncommon liver cystic lesion, with only 100 cases being published. [104–108] It is postulated that CHFC derives from intrahepatic embryonic remnants that differentiate towards respiratory tissue rather than biliary. [6, 105–107, 109]

It is usually benign, solitary, single, subcapsular and unilocular, and is often located in segment IV. It is of variable size, but usually under 4 cm. [104–111] Its content is viscous or mucoid. [104, 106, 108, 109] The mean age of onset is 48 years with a slight predominance towards men. [104, 105, 110] Histologically, there are 4 layers: mucin-producing pseudostratified ciliated columnar epithelium, subepithelial connective tissue, stroma, and fibrous capsule. [6, 105, 107–109, 111] Three cases of squamous cell carcinoma in CHFC that developed in previous squamous metaplasia foci have been described, suggesting a progression from dysplasia to carcinoma. [104, 105, 111–113]

Its diagnosis is usually incidental because they are asymptomatic in 80% of cases. [104–106, 108, 110] The most typical symptom is abdominal pain, although it can also cause jaundice or portal hypertension. [104–108, 111, 112]

On the ultrasound image, it appears as an anechoic or hypoechoic, well-defined, round lesion, with a visible intracystic echogenic mass. [104, 110] The CT image shows hypodense lesions without contrast enhancement. On MRI, the T2 hyperintensity is characteristic, with a variable T1 intensity depending on the content. [104, 106–109, 111] Puncturing has a positive predictive value of 76%. [104]

The traditional treatment was puncturing with aspiration or injection of sclerosing agents, with surgical treatment recommended only in symptomatic lesions with uncertain diagnosis. [106, 107] Publication of 3 cases of malignisation (3% of the total) raises doubts about the most appropriate treatment. [106, 111, 112] CHFC must always be resected if larger than 4 cm (the 3 patients with large cysts had malignant CHFC), symptomatic, with progressive growth or when there is a mass on the cyst wall. [104, 106, 111] Complete laparoscopic resection of CHFC is an interesting option. [111]

Caroli Disease

Patients with Caroli Disease have not real liver cysts, but classically are included in reviews about liver cysts.

In 1958, Jacques Caroli first described a cavernous biliary ectasia now known as Caroli disease (CD). [114-116] CD is a congenital condition with autosomal recessive inheritance characterized by absent or abnormal embryological bile duct modeling. CD gives rise to multifocal saccular nonobstructive dilatation of the intrahepatic large bile ducts and presents clinically with recurrent cholangitis. [114-121] About 21% of patients exhibit diffuse biliary dilation without sacculations. [116] CD is characterized by pure ectasia of the bile ducts without fibrosis or other concomitant histological lesions. [118.120] It is included in the classification of cystic dilatation of the bile duct as Type 5 and represents 1% of these lesions. [114, 118, 119, 122, 123] There are two forms of CD: Type 1, occasionally bilobar but more often monolobar, and Type 2, also called Caroli syndrome, consisting of diffuse bilobar involvement associated with liver fibrosis. [114, 117, 118, 121] CD is associated with polycystic kidney disease. CD can affect a single lobe in 15-20% of cases. [114, 115, 118, 120] Unilobar CD affects the left lobe in 80% of cases. In 25% of cases, patients are seen at an age over 50 years and gallstones are present in 43%. [114-117, 120, 121, 124]

The diagnosis of CD is based on imaging methods. Abdominal ultrasound is the most cost-effective method for identifying dilatation of the intrahepatic bile ducts up to 1-2 mm and hepatolithiasis. CT has a sensitivity of 63-81% for the diagnosis of hepatolithiasis, detecting hypointense cysts connected to the bile duct. [116] On MR, the lesions manifest as hypointense images on T1 and hyperintense on T2, corresponding to dilated and obstructed saccular intrahepatic bile ducts that communicate with the bile duct. Ultrasonography and intraoperative cholangiography are important in confirming the diagnosis and planning surgery.

The differential diagnosis of CD includes primary sclerosing cholangitis, recurrent cholangitis, polycystic liver disease and biliary papillomatosis. Recurrent cholangitis is difficult to distinguish radiologically from the diffuse form of CD. [116]

Bile stagnation occurs in CD and there is a high incidence of cholangitis and liver abscess, originating hepatolithiasis and biliary sepsis. [116-118, 121] Portal hypertension and biliary cirrhosis may develop. In addition, the repeated inflammatory processes can cause the development of cholangiocarcinoma in CD (7-14% of patients). [116-118, 121, 124]

Nonsurgical treatments, such as treatment with ursodeoxycholic acid, are not curative. Surgical options include the surgical removal of stones without resection, but it is accompanied by a high rate of gallstone recurrence. The treatment of choice for monolobar CD is lobar hepatectomy because it is a definitive solution for the problem. [114, 117-119, 121, 123] In the case of bilobar CD or CD associated with portal fibrosis and portal hypertension, secondary biliary cirrhosis and untreatable septic complications may be present and the possibility of liver transplantation must be weighed. [114, 117-119, 121, 123]

Other Rare Cystic Lesions

Other rare cystic lesions have been described:

- Intrahepatic pancreatic pseudocyst: only 27 cases were described up to 2006. They are usually located in the left hepatic lobe, are usually asymptomatic, and diagnosis is incidental. Diagnostic confirmation comes after puncture when there is a fluid rich in amylase. [125]Treatment ranges from monitoring and percutaneous drainage to surgery; [125]

- Post-traumatic cysts: the conservative management of liver injuries has increased the number of post-traumatic cysts. Only those symptomatic ones or those with diagnostic uncertainty should be operated on; [1, 5, 7, 126]
- Hamartomas: also called von Meyenburg complexes. They are caused by a failure of involution of the embryonic bile ducts. [126] They are multiple lesions of 0.1–1.5 cm and are not communicated with the bile duct. [127] Autopsy incidence varies between 0% and 2.8%. They are usually incidental findings, as they are usually asymptomatic but may exceptionally cause microabscesses or degenerate into cholangiocarcinoma. [127, 128] A CT image may be confused with multiple liver metastases but MRI provides an accurate diagnosis; [127]
- Epidermoid cyst;
- Lymphangiomas;
- Biloma: These are caused by spontaneous, traumatic or iatrogenic rupture of the biliary system;
- Biliary intraductal papillary mucinous tumour: There are 2 types, cystic and non-cystic. [101]

REFERENCES

[1]   Mazza OM; Fernandez DL Pekolj J, Pfaffen G, Sanchez R, Molmenti E, Santibañes E., Management of non parasitic hepatic cysts; *J. Am Coll Surg* 2009; 209:733-739.

[2]   Erdogan D., Van Delden O.M., Rauws E. J., Busch O. R. C., Lameris J.S., Gouma D. J., Van Guilk T. M, Results of percutaneous sclerotherapy and surgical treatment in patients with symptomatic simple liver cysts and polycystic liver disease, *World J. Gastroenterol* 2007; 13: 3095-3100.

[3]   Regev A, Reddy KR, Berho M Sleeman D, Levi JU, Livingstone AS et al, Large cystic lesions of the liver in adults: a 15-year experience in a tertiary center, *J. Am Coll Surg* 2001; 193:36-45.

[4]   Marcos R, Rodriguez A, Martin J, Ramos P, Galvan M, Gutierrez A et al Cistoadenomas hepatobiliares, *Cir Esp* 2006; 79: 375-8.

[5]   Cowles R. A., Mulhouland M. W.,Solitary hepatic cysts, *J. Am Coll Surg* 2000; 191:311-321.

[6]   Hansman M.F., Ryan J. A. J., Holmes J. H., Hogan S., Lee F. T., Kramer D., Biehl T., Management and long term follow-up of hepatic cysts, *Am J. Surg* 2001; 181: 404-410.

[7]   Lin C. C., Lin S. C., Ko W. C., Chang K. M., Shih S. C.,Adenocarcinoma and infection in a solitary hepatic cyst, *World J Gastroenterol* 2005; 11: 1881-1883.

[8]   Poggi G., Gatti C., Delmonte A., Teragni C., Bernardo G., Spontaneous rupture of non-parasitic hepatic cyst, *Int J Clin Pract* 2006; 60: 99-103.

[9]   Miyamoto M., Oka M., Izumiya T., Nagaoka T., Ishihara Y., Udea K. et al, Non parasitic cyst giant hepatic cyst Rausing obstructive jaundice was successfully treated with monoethanolamine oleate, *Intern Med* 2006; 45:621-625.

[10]   Frider B., Alvarez J., Chiappeta L., Amante M., Non parasitic symple liver cyst: always a benign entity? Unusual presentation of a cystadenoma, *Dig. Dis. Sci* 2005;50:317-319.

[11]   Klingler P.J., Gadenstatter M., Schmid T., Bodner E., Schwelberger H.G., Treatment of hepatic cysts in the era of laparoscopic surgery, *Br. J. Surg.* 1997; 84: 438-444.

[12]   Zhang Y. L., Yuan L., Shen F., Wang Y.,Hemorrhagic hepatic cysts mimicking biliary cystadenoma, *World J Gastroenterol* 2009; 28: 4601-4603.

[13]   Garcea G., Pattenden C. J., Stephenson J., Dennison A. R., Berry D. P., Nine-year single center experience with nonparasitic liver cysts: diagnosis and Management, *Dig Dis Sci* 2007; 52. 185-191.

[14]   Petri A., Hohn J., Makula E., Kokai E. L., Savanya G. K., Boros M., Balogh A. Experience with different methods of treatment of nonparasitic liver cysts, *Langenbecks Arch Surg.* 2002; 387:229-233.

[15]   Van Sonnenberg E., Wroblicka J.T., D´Agostino H.B., Mathieson J. R., Casola G., O´Laoide R., Cooperberg P. L., Symptomatic hepatic cysts: percutaneous drainage and sclerosis, *Radiology* 1994; 190:387-392.

[16]   Loehe F., Globke B., Marnoto R., Bruns C. J., Graeb C., Winter H. et al.Long term results alter surgical treatmetn of nonparasitic hepatic cysts, *Am J. Surg* 2010; 200:23-31.

[17]   Treckmann J. W., Paul A., Sgourakis G., Heuer M., Wandelt M., Sotiropoulos G. C., Surgical treatment of nonparasitic cysts of the liver: open versus laparoscopic treatment, *Am J. Surg* 2010; 199: 776-781.

[18]   Laparoscopic excision of a large hepatic cyst, Tabrizian P., Midulla P. S. *JSLS.* 2010 Apr-Jun;14(2):272-4.

[19]   Buyse S., Asselah T., Vilgrain V., Parais V., Sauvanet A., Consigny Y. et al Acute pulmonary embolism: a rare complication of a large non parasitic hepatic cyst; *Eur J Gastroenterol Hepatol* 2004; 16: 1241-1244.

[20]   Thomas K. T., Welch D., Trueblood A., Sulur P., Wise P., Gorden D. L. et al, Effective treatment of biliary cystadenoma, *Ann Surg* 2005; 241: 769-773.

[21]   Pitale A., Bohra A. K., Diamond T. Management of symptomatic liver cysts; *Ulster Med J* 2002;71:106-110.

[22]   Pons F., Llovet J. M., Actitud a seguir ante una lesión hepática focal; *Rev Esp Enf Digest* 2004; 96:567-577.

[23]   Farges O., Bismuth H., Fenestration in the management of polycystic liver disease. *World J Surg* 1995;19:25-30.

[24]   Bai X. L., Liang T. B., Yu J., Wang W. L., Shen Y., Zhang M., Zheng S. S., Long term results of laparoscopic fenestration for patients with congenital liver cysts, *Hepatobiliary Pancreat Dis Int* 2007; 6:600-603.

[25]   Gigot J., F., Legrand M., Hubens G., Canniere L., Wibin E., Deweer F. et al, Laparoscopc treatment of nonparasitic liver cysts: adequate selection of patients ad surgical technique, *World J. Surg* 1996; 556-561.

[26]   Palanivelu C., Rangarajan M., Senthilkumar R., Mdankumar M. V., Laparoscopic management of symptomatic multiple hepatic cysts: a combination of deroofing and radical excision, *JSLS* 2007; 11:466-469.

[27]   Gambin T. C., Holloway S. E., Heckman J. T., Geller D. A., Laparoscopic resection of benign hepatic cysts: a new standard, *J Am Coll Surg* 2008; 207:731-736.

[28] Tocchi A., Mazzoni G., Costa G., Cassini D., Bettelli E., Agostini N., Miccini M., Symptomatic nonparasitic hepatic cysts, *Arch Surg* 2002; 137:154-158.

[29] Yoshida H., Onda M., Tajiri T., Mamada Y., Taniai N., Uchida E. et al., Spontaneous disappearance of a hepatic cyst, *J Nippon Med Sch* 2001;68: 58-60.

[30] Nagorney D. M., Surgical management of cystic disease of the liver pp 1261-1276. *Surgery of the liver and biliary tract*; 4ª Ed. WB Saunders Ed. L Blumgart 2007.

[31] Krakenbuhl L., Baer H. U., Renzulli P., Z'graggen K., Frei E., Buchler M., Laparoscopic management of nonparasitic syptom-producing solitary hepatic cysts, *J Am Coll Surg* 1996; 183: 493-498.

[32] Kitajima Y., Okayama Y., Hirai M., Hayashi K., Imai H., Okamoto T et al, Intracystic hemorrhage of a simple liver cyst mimicking a biliary cystadenocarcinoma, *J Gastroenterol* 2003; 38:190-193.

[33] Van Keipema L., Drenth J. P., *Effect of octreotide on polycystic liver* volume, Liver Int 2009; 633-634.

[34] Salemis N.S., Georgoulis E., Gourgiotis S., Tsohataridis E., Spontaneous rupture of a giant non parasitic hepatic cyst presenting as an acute abdomen, *Ann Hepatol* 2007; 6:190-193.

[35] Leung T.K., Lee C. M., Chen H. C., Fatal thrombotic complcations of hepatic cystic compression of the inferior vena: a case report. *World J Gastroenterol* 2005; 11:1728-1729.

[36] Macho O., Gomez J., Nuñez A., Narvaiza L., Albeniz L., Giant simple hepatic cyst as dyspnea symptoma in a 93 year-old patient, *An Med Interna* 2007; 24:135-137.

[37] Takahashi G., Yoshida H., Mamada Y., Taniai N., Bando K., Tajiri T., Intracystic hemorrhage of a large simple hepatic cyst, *J Nippon Med Sch* 2008; 75:302-305.

[38] Alfonso R., Melo F., Ballester J. M., Caro F., Sarcoma pleomórfico hepático sobre quiste hepático no parasitario, *Cir Esp* 2009;86:386-387.

[39] Kim H. S., Kim G. Y., Lim S. J., Lee S. M., Kim Y. W.,Undifferentiated pleomorphic sarcoma of the liver presenting as a unilocular cyst, *Hepatobiliary Pancreat Dis Int* 2009; 8:541-543.

[40] Naganuma H., Funaoka M., Fujimori S., Ishida H., Komatsuda T., Yamada M et al, Hepatic cyst with intracystic bleeding: contrast-enhanced sonographic findings, *J Med Ultrasonics* 2006; 33:105-107.

[41] Hsieh C. B., Chen C. J., Yu J. C., Chang T. M., Gao H. W., Primary squamous cell carcinoma of the liver arising from a complex liver cyst: report of a case, *Surg Today* 2005; 35:328-331.

[42] Giuliante F., D'Acapito F., Vellone M., Giovannini I., Nuzzo G., Risk of laparoscopic fenestration of liver cysts, *Surg Endosc* 2003; 17:1735-1738.

[43] Madariaga J. R., Iwatsuki S., Starzl T., Todo S., Selby R., Zetti G., Hepatic resection for cystic lesions of the liver, *Ann Surg* 1993; 218: 610-614

[44] Konstadoulakis M., Gomatos I. P., Albanopoulos K., Alexakis N., Leandros E., Laparoscopic fenestration for the treatment of patients with sever adult polycystic liver disease, *Am J Surg* 2003; 189. 71-75.

[45] Yang G. S., Li Q. G., Lu J. H., Yang N., Zhang H. B., Zhou X. P., Combined hepatic resection with fenestration for highly symptomatic polycystic liver disease: a report on seven patients, *World J Gastroenterol* 2004;10: 2598-2601.

[46] Gagner M., Rogula T., Selzer D., Laparoscopic liver resection: benefits and controversies, *Surg Clin N Am* 2004; 84: 451-462.

[47] Fiamingo P., Tedeschi U., Veroux M., Cillo U., Brolese A., Da Rold A., Madia C., Zanus G., D'Amico D.F., Laparoscopic treatment of simple hepatic cysts and polycystic liver disease, *Surg Endosc* 2003 Apr;17(4):623-6.

[48] Aoki T., Kato T., Yasuda D., Shimizu Y., Murai N., Sato A. et al, Cyst wall resection and ablation by hand- assisted laparoscopic surgery combined with argon plasma coagulator for huge hepatic cysts, *Int Surg* 2007; 92:.361-366.

[49] Du X. L., Ma Q. J., Wu T., Lu J. G., Bao G. Q., Chu Y. K., Treatment of hepatic cysts by B-ultrasound-guided radiofrequency ablation, *Hepatobiliary Pancreat Dis Int* 2007; 6:330-332.

[50] Russel R. T., Pinson C. W., Surgical Management of polycystic liver disease, *World J Gastroenterol* 2007; 13: 5052-5059.

[51] Bistritz L., Tamboli C., Bigam D., Bain V. G., Polycystic liver disease: experience at a teaching hospital, *Am J Gastroenterol* 2005; 100:2212-2227.

[52] Li T. J., Zhang H. B., Lu J. H., Zhao J., Yang N., Yang G. S., Treatment of polycystic liver disease with resection-fenestration and a new classification, *World J Gastroenterol* 2008; 14:5066-5072.

[53] Grams J., Teh S. H., Torres V. E., Andrews J. C., Nagorney D. M., Inferior vena cava stenting: a safe and effective treatment for intractable ascites in patients with polycystic liver disease, *J Gastrointest Surg* 2007; 11:985-990.

[54] Varona J. F., Usandizaga I., Perez Maestu R., Marcos J., Lozano F., Varón de 77 años con ictericia y prurito, *Rev Clin Esp* 2006; 206:197-198.

[55] Lang H., Woellwarth J. V., Oldhafer K. J., Behrend M., Schlitt H. J., Nashan B., Pichlmayr R., Liver transplantation in patients with polycystic liver disease, *Transplant Proc* 1997; 29: 2832-2833.

[56] Chavez R. E., Jamieson N. V., *Poliquistosis hepática* pp 88-89. Trasplante hepático. 1ªEd Editorial Elba. J. Berenguer, P Parrilla 1999.

[57] Vall Llovera J., Bosch A., Gil E., Pons L., Barba S., Palau M. et al, Poliquistosis hepática del adulto abscesificada, *Cir Esp* 2002; 72:113-115.

[58] Waanders E., Van Keimpema L., Brouwer J.T., Van Oijen M.G.H., Aerts R, Sweep F.G.C.J .et al, CA19-9 is extremely elevated in polycystic liver disease, *Liver Int* 2009; 1389-1395.

[59] Barahona J., Camacho J., Cerda E., Hernández J., Yamamoto J.K., Torre A., Uribe M., Factors that influence outcome in non-invasive and invasive treatment in polycystic liver disease patients, *World J Gastroenterol* 2008; 14: 3195-3200.

[60] Morgan D. E., Lockhart M. E., Canon C. L., Holcombe M. P., Bynon J. S. Polycystic liver disease: multimodality Imaging for complications and transplant evaluation, *Radiographics* 2006; 26: 1655-1668.

[61] Parks R.W., Garden O.J., *Benign liver lesions* pp 75-105. Hepatobiliary and pancreatic Surgery 4Ed W.B, Saunders E.D., O.J. Garden 2010.

[62] Aussilhou B., Doufle G., Hubert C., Francoz C., Paugam C., Paradis V. et al, Extended liver resection for polycystic liver disease can challenge liver transplantation, *Ann Surg* 2010; 252: 735-743.

[63] Pirenne J., Aerts R., Yoong K., Gunson B., Koshiba T. et al, Liver transplantation for polycystic liver disease, *Liver Transpl* 2001; 7: 238-245.

[64] Van Keimpema L., Nevens F., Vanslembrouck R., Van Oijen M.G.H., Hoffmann A.L., Dekker H.M., De Man R.A., Drenth J.P., Lanreotide reduces the volumen of polycystic liver: a randomized double-blind, placeb-controlled trial, *Gastroenterology* 2009, 137:1661-1668.

[65] Hoevenaren I.,A., Wester R., Schrier R.W., McFann K., Doctor R.B., Drenth J.P., et al, Polycystic liver: Clinical characteristics of patients with isolated polycystic liver disease compared with patients with polycystic liver and autosomal dominant polycystic kidney disease, *Liver Int.*

[66] Van Keimpema L., Hockerstedt K., Treatment of polycystic liver disease, *Br J Surg* 2007; 96:1379-1380.

[67] Swenson K, Seu P, Kinkhabwala M, Maggard M, Martin P et al.,Liver Transplantation for adult polycystic liver disease, *Hepatology* 1998; 28:412-415.

[68] Jones R.S., Surgical management of non-parasitic liver cysts pp1211-1217; *Surgery of the liver and biliary tract,* 4ª Ed. WB Saunders Ed. L Blumgart 2007.

[69] Iglesias D.M., Palmitano J.A., Arrizurieta E., Kornblihtt A.R., Herrera M., Bernath V., Martin R.S.,Isolated polycystic liver disease not linked to polycystic kidney disease 1 and 2, *Dig Dis Sci* 1999 Feb; 44(2): 385-8.

[70] Reynolds D.M., Falk C.T., Li A., King B.F., Kamath P.S. et al, Identification of a locus for autosomal dominant polycystic liver disease on chromosome 19 p 13.2-13.1, *Am J Hum Genet* 2000; 1598-1604.

[71] Arnold H.L., Harrison S.A.,New advances in evaluation and management of patients with polycystic liver disease, *Am J Gastroenterol* 2005; 100:2569-2582.

[72] Gustafsson B.I., Friman S., Mjornstedt L., Olausson M., Backman L., Liver transplantation for polycystic liver disease: indications and outcome, *Transplant Proc* 2003; 35:813-814.

[73] Schnelldorfer T., Torres V.E., Zakaria S., Rosen C.E., Nagorney D.M., Polycycstic liver disease. A critical appraisal of hepatic resection, cyst fenestration and liver transplantation, *Ann Surg* 2009; 250:112-118.

[74] Van Keimpema L., Ruurda J.P., Ernst M.F., Van Geffen H.J.A.A., Drenth J.P.H., Laparoscopic fenestration of liver cysts in polycystic liver disease results in a median volumen reduction of 12.5%, *J Gastrointest Surg* 2008; 12:477-482.

[75] Di Carlo I., Di Stefano A., Pulvirenti E., Toro A., Laparoscopic excision of a case of percutaneous cystohepatic fistula in a patient affected by polycystic disease of the liver: point of technique, *Surg Laparosc Endosc Percutan Tech* 2008; 18:514-5.

[76] Starzl T., Reyes J., Tzakis A., Mieles L., Todo S., Gordon R., Liver Transplantation for polycystic liver disease, *Arch Surg* 1990; 125: 575-577.

[77] Gigot J.F., Jadoul P., Que F., Van Beers B.E., eienne J, Horsmans Y. et al, Adult polycystic liver disease: is fenestration the most adequate operation for long term management? *Ann Surg* 1997; 225:286-294.

[78] Nakaoka R., Das K., Kudo M., Chung H., Innoue T., Percutaneous aspirationand ethanolamine oleate sclerotherapy for sustained resolution of symptomatic polycystic lver disease: an initial experience, *AJR* 2009; 193:1540-5.

[79] Kwok M.K., Lewin K.J., Massive hepatomegaly in adult polycystic liver disease, *Am J Surg Pathol* 1998; 12:321-324.

[80]   Ramia J.M., San Juan F., Orbis J.F., Moya A., Lopez-Andujar R., De Juan M., Mir J., Tratamiento de la poliquistosis hepatica mediante transplante hepatico; *Cir Esp.* 2004, 76 (6), 358-62.

[81]   Jeyarajah D. R., Gonwa T.A., Testa G., Abbasoglu O., Goldstein R. et al, Liver and Kidney transplantation for polycystic disease, *Transplantation* 1998; 66:529-531.

[82]   Koyama I., Fuchinoue S., Urashima Y., Kato Y., Tsuji K et al, Living related liver transplantation for polycystic liver disease, *Transpl Int* 2002; 15: 578-80.

[83]   Teoh A.Y.B., Ng S.S.M., Lee K.F., Lai P.B.S., Biliary cystoadenoma and other complicated cystic lesions of the liver: diagnostic and therapeutic challenges, *World J Surg* 2006; 30: 1560-1566.

[84]   Manouras A., Markogiannakis H., Lagoudianakis E., Katergiannakis V., Biliary cystadenoma with mesenchynal stroma: report of a case and review of the literature, *World J Gastroenterol* 2006; 12: 6062-6069.

[85]   Yu F.C., Chen J.H., Yang K.C., Wu C.C., Chou Y.Y., Hepatobiliary cystadenoma: a report of two cases. *J Gastrointest Liver Dis* 2008; 17:203-206.

[86]   Fukunaga N., Ishikawa M., Ishikura H., Ichimori T., Kimura S., Sakata A et al, Hepatobiliary cystadenoma exhibiting morphologic changes from simple hepatic cyst shown by 11-year follow up imagings, *World J Surg Oncol* 2008; 6:129-135.

[87]   Ramirez C., Ruiz M., Santoyo J., Iaria M., Suarez M., Jimenez M. et al, Cistoadenoma biliar con estroma mesenquimal "ovarian like" y niveles elevados de CA19.9, *Rev Esp Enf Dig* 2004; 96:588-589.

[88]   Den Hoed P.T., Lameris H., Klooswijk B., Ijzermans J.N.M., Biliary cystadenoma: an uncommon cause of cholestatic jaundice, *Eur J Surg Oncol* 1999;25:335-6.

[89]   Catinis G. E., Frey D. J., Sinner J. W., Balart L. A., Hepatic cystadenoma: an unusual presentation; *Am J. Gastroenterol* 1998; 93: 827-829.

[90]   Dixon E., Sutherland F.R., Mitchell P., McKinnon G., Nayak V., Cystadenomas of the liver: a spectrum disease, *Can J. Surg* 2001; 44: 371-375.

[91]   Beuran M., Dan Venter M., Dumitru L.,Large mucinous biliary cystadenoma with "ovarian-like" stroma: a case report, *World J. Gastroenterol* 2006; 12:3779-3781.

[92]   Fiamingo P., Veroux M., Cillo U., Basso S., Buffone A., D´Amico D. F.,Incidental cystadenoma after laparoscopic treatment of hepatic cysts: which strategy; *Surg Laparosc Endosc Percutan Tech* 2004; 14: 282-284.

[93]   Vogt D. P., Henderson J. M., Chmielewski E., Cystadenoma and cystadenocarcinoma of the liver: a single center experience; *J. Am Coll Surg* 2005; 200:727-733.

[94]   Pojchamarnwiputh S., Na Chiangmai W., Chotirosniramit A., Lertprasertsuke N., Computed tomography of biliary cystadenoma and biliary cystadenocarcinoma; *Singapore Med J.* 2008; 49: 392-396.

[95]   Buetow P. C., Buck J. L., Pantongrag-Brown L., Ros P. R., Devaney K., Goodman Z., Cruess D. F., Biliary cystoadenoma and cystoadenocarcinoma: Clinical-Imaging-Pathologic correlation with emphasis on the importante of ovarian stroma; *Radiology* 1995; 196: 805-810.

[96]   Zhou J. P., Dong M., Zhang Y., Kong F. M., Guo K. J, Tian Y. L., Giant mucinous biliary cystadenoma: a case report; *Hepatobiliary Panceat Dis Int* 2007; 6:101-103.

[97]   Wheleer D. A., Edmondson H. A., Cystadenoma with mesenchymal stroma in the liver and the bile ducts. A clinicopathologic study of 17 cases*; Cancer* 1985; 56: 1434-1445.

[98] Daniels J. A., Coad J. E., Payne W., Kosari K., Sielaff T. D., Biliary cystoadenomas: hormone receptor expresión and clinical management; *Dig Dis Sci* 2006; 51:623-628.

[99] Lauffer J. M., Baer H. U., Maurer CA, Stoupis C, Zimmerman A, Buchler M.W., Biliary cystoadenocarcinoma of the liver: the need for compelte resection. *Eur J Cancer* 1998; 34: 1845-1851.

[100] Lim J. H., Jang K. T., Rhim H., Kim Y. S., Lee K. T., Choi S. H., Biliary cystic intraductal papillary mucinous tumor and cystadenoma/cystadenocarcinoma differentiation by CT; *Abdom Imaging* 2007; 32:644-651.

[101] Koffron A., Ferrario M., Rao S, Abecassis M., Intrahepatic biliary cystadenoma: role of cyst fluid analysis and surgical management in the laparoscopic era; *Surgery* 2004; 136: 926-36.

[102] Horsmans Y., Laka A., Gigot J.P., Geubel A.P., Serum and cystic fluid CA19-9 determinations as a diagnostic help in liver cysts of uncertain nature; *Liver* 1996; 16: 255-257.

[103] Sharma S., Dean A.G., Corn A., Kohli V., Wright H., Sebastian A., Jabbour N.,Ciliated hepatic foregut cyst: an increasingly diagnosed condition ; *Hepatobiliary Pancreat Dis* 2008; 7: 581-589.

[104] Ben Mena N., Zalinski S., Svrcek M., Lewin M., Fléjou J.F., Wendum D, Paye F.,Ciliated hepatic foregut cyst with extensive squamous metaplasia: report of a case Virchows; *Arch* 2006; 449: 730-733.

[105] Kiyochi H, Okada K, Iwakawa K, Nakanisshi M, Satoh H, Iimori S et al Ciliated hepatic foregut cyst with obstructive jaundice; *Case Rep Gastroenterol* 2008; 2: 479-485.

[106] Fernandez L, Nuño J, García-Moreno F, Lopez-Hervas P, Quijano Y, Mena A et al Quiste hepatico ciliado embrionario multilocular. Aportación de un nuevo caso y revisión de la literatura, *Rev Esp Enf Dig* 2005; 97: 606-608.

[107] Shaw J. M., Krige J. E. J., Beningfield S. J., Locketz M.L., Ciliated hepatic foregut cyst: a rare cystic liver lesion, *J Gastrointest Surg* 2008; 12: 1304-1305.

[108] Straus T, Osipov V., Ciliated hepatic foregut cyst in a patient with renal cell carcinoma BMC; *Cancer* 2006; 6: 244-250.

[109] Fang S.H., Dong D.J., Zhang S.Z., Imaging features of ciliated hepatic foregut cyst; *World J Gastroenterol*; 2005; 11: 4287–9. 111.

[110] Hirata M, Ishida H, Konno K, Nishiura S., Ciliated hepatic foregut cyst: case report with an emphasis on US findings; *Abdom Imaging* 2001; 26: 594–6.

[111] Goodman M.D., Mak G.Z., Reynolds J.P., Tevar A.D., Pritts T.A., Laparoscopic excision of a ciliated hepatic foregut cyst; *JSL.* 2009; 13: 96–100.

[112] Furlanetto A, Palo dei Tois A., Squamous cell carcinoma arising in a ciliated hepatic foregut cyst; *Virchows Arch* 2002; 441: 296–8.

[113] Kassahun WT, Kahn T, Wittekind C, Mossner J, Caca K, Hauss J, Lamesch P., Caroli´s disease: liver resection and liver transplantation. Experience in 33 patients; *Surgery* 2005; 138: 888-898.

[114] Garre C, Mercader J, García B, Saez R, Albadalejo A, Baños R., Enfermedad de Caroli segmentaria; Rev Esp Enferm Dig 2002; 94:504-505.

[115] Levy A., Rohrmann C.A., Murakata L.A., Lonergan G.J.,Caroli´s disease: radiologic spectrum with pathologic correlation. AJR 2002; 179:1053-1057.

[116] Bockhorn M, Malago M, Lang H, Nadalin S, Paul A, Saner F et al, The role of surgery in Caroli´s Disease, J Am Coll Surg 2006; 202:928-932.

[117] Medrano R, Artigas V, Sancho F.J., Marin G., Rodriguez M., Trias M., Hepatectomía parcial curativa en la enfermedad de Caroli del adulto; *Cir Esp;* 2007; 81:218-221.

[118] Mabrut JY, Bozio G, Hubert C, Gigot J.F., Management of congenital bile duct cysts; *Dig Surg* 2010; 27:12-18.

[119] Escartín P., Patología de la placa ductal; *Gastroenterol Hepatol* 1998; 21:492-497.

[120] Ulrich P, Pratschke J, Pascher A, Neumann U.P., Lopez E., Jonas S., Neuhaus P.; Long term outcome of liver resection and transplantation for Caroli disease and syndrome. *Ann Surg* 2008; 247. 357-363.

[121] Soreide K, Korner H, Havnen J, Soreide J.A., Bile duct cysts in adults Br J Surg 2004; 91:1538-1548.

[122] Dominguez E., Dilataciones cóngenitas de la via biliar; *Cir Esp* 2010; 88:285-291.

[123] Gillet M., Favre S., Fontolliet C., Halkic N., Mantion G., Heyd B.; Monolobar Caroli disease. Apropos of 12 cases. *Chirurgie* 1999; 124:13-18.

[124] Les I, Córdoba J., Vargas V., Guarner L., Boyé R., Pineda V.Pseudoquiste pancreático de localización hepatica; *Rev Esp Enferm Dig* 2006; 98:616-620.

[125] Chen B.K., Gamagami R.A., Kang J., Easter D., Lopez T., Symptomatic post-traumatic cyst of the liver: treatment by laparoscopic surgery; *J Lap* Adv Surg Tech 2001; 11:41-42.

[126] Martin D.R., Kalb B., Sarmiento J.M., Heffron T.G., Coban I., Adsay N.V., Giant and complicated variants of cystic bile duct harmatomas of the liver: MRI finding and pathological correlation, *J Magn reson Imaging* 2010; 31:903-911.

[127] Rocken C., Pross M., Brucks U., Ridwelski K., Roessner A., Cholangiocarcinoma occurring in a liver with multiple bile duct hamartomas, *Arch Pathol Lab Med* 2000; 124:1704-6.

Chapter 6

CAUSES AND DIAGNOSIS OF CYSTS

Babatunde O. Akinbami[1] and Olufemi G. Omitola

Department of Oral & Maxillofacial Surgery and Department of Oral Pathology & Oral
Biology, University of Port Harcourt,
Choba, Rivers State, Nigeria

ABSTRACT

Cysts of the oral cavity are relatively a common lesion which the oral surgeon and general dentist will have to manage during their practice. Head and neck cysts are generally a benign lesion with history of slow growth and may be asymptomatic except when they increase in size and also become secondarily infected. However, some odontogenic cyst have been reported to be aggressive especially the parakeratinized type of odontogenic keratocyst. This is one of the reasons why it was recently classified as a tumor. Also more sinister conditions like ameloblastoma, squamous cell and mucoepidermoid carcinoma have been reported to arise from the wall of a cyst. Our experience has shown that most of the initial histological diagnoses of cysts obtained from small tissues taken during incision biopsies are not very dependable and misleading to the surgeons as some of these lesions eventually turn out to be unicystic ameloblastoma after histological processing of post-operative specimens. Cyst linings must always be sent for histopathological examination after surgery.

It is therefore important that a dentist have a good knowledge of these important conditions so as to be able to make an accurate diagnosis and then institute an appropriate referral.

CHAPTER INTRODUCTION

A cyst is a pathological cavity that may or not be lined by epithelium and filled with gas, fluid or semi-solid. Many classifications exist but the most recent 2004 World Health Organization classification gives an elaborate categorization of all cysts affecting the maxillofacial region.

---

[1] E-mail address: akinbamzy3@yahoo.com

I. CYSTS OF THE JAWS

A) Epithelial (True Cyst)

a) Odontogenic
    Inflammatory

- radicular cyst (apical / lateral)
- residual cyst
- paradental cyst
- inflammatory collateral cyst

Developmental

- gingival cysts of infants
- gingival cyst of adults
- primordial cyst
- odontogenic keratocyst and Gorlin-Goltz syndrome
- dentigerous (follicular) cyst
- eruption cyst
- lateral periodontal cyst
- botryoid odontogenic cysts
- glandular odontogenic (sialo-odontogenic / mucoepidermoid-odontogenic) cyst
- calcifying odontogenic cyst

b) Non-odontogenic

- naso-palatine duct (incisive canal) cyst
- naso-labial (naso-alveolar) cyst
- midpalatine raphae cyst of infants
- median palatine,
- median alveolar and median mandibular cysts
- globulomaxillary cyst; possibly gone into extinction, now exist as globulomaxillary lesion.

B) Non-epithelial (False Cyst)

- solitary (traumatic /simple/haemorrhagic) bone cyst
- aneurysmal bone cyst
- static bone cyst (Stafne's Idiopathic bone cyst)

II. Cysts Associated with the Maxillary Antrum

- benign mucosal cyst of the maxillary antrum
- post-operative maxillary cyst (surgical ciliated cyst of the maxilla)

III. Cysts of the Soft Tissues of the Mouth, Face and Neck

- dermoid and epidermoid cyst
- lymphoepithelial (branchial cleft) cyst
- thyroglossal duct cyst
- cystic hygroma
- anterior median lingual cyst (intralingual cyst of fore-gut origin)
- oral cyst with gastric / intestinal epithelium (oral alimentary tract cyst)
- naso-pharyngeal cysts
- thymic cysts
- cysts of salivary gland
- mucous extravasation cyst
- mucous retention cyst
- polycystic (degenerative) disease of parotid gland
- parasitic cysts (hydatid cyst cysticerus cellulosae trichinosis)

Other classifications by Robinson (1945), Kruger (1964), Lucas (1964) and Gorlin (1970) do not give a comprehensive description which should include cysts of the sinuses and those affecting the soft tissues.

Aetiology and General Principles of Management

Causes of these cysts from the classification are broadly related to inflammation, from trauma and infections or developmental from minor to major genetic mutilations. Various theories have been proposed for initiation, formation and maturation of these cysts.

Most of the cysts do not give any symptom or sign during the initial phase; they can only be found on a routine clinical or radiological evaluation.

Diagnosis of Cyst:

Oral Cysts should be suspected when-

1. The swelling is found to be smooth, rounded and painless expansion of the jaw bone
2. The teeth in relation to the cyst may be missing in younger patients; a dentigerous or primordial cyst is suspected
3. Completely missing tooth in the alveolar bone or mouth is usually due to primordial cyst while absent tooth in the mouth but present in the alveolar bone; is due to dentigerous cyst

4. Mobility of teeth may be due to dentigerous or odontogenic keratocyst due to bone resorption rarely does radicular cyst cause mobility
5. The swelling is in relation to a non-vital, carious or fractured tooth; a radicular cyst may be suspected. In older patients, clinical absence of the non-vital tooth with a history of extraction leads to the diagnosis of residual cyst
6. The swellings are painful and tender swellings may indicate an infected cyst
7. Keratocyst or primordial cyst may present as slow or moderately fast growing hard swelling, anteroposterior growth from the angle of the mandible, producing facial asymmetry. Later produce buccolingual expansion

Cysts of the soft tissues of the head and neck are mostly found in children, though some occur in young adults

Ranulas actually are clinical .diagnosis which refer generally to any swelling in the floor of the mouth, and they include the oral cysts caused by the rupture of a salivary gland duct from trauma, resulting in collection of the saliva in the surrounding connective tissues; extravasation phenomenon- this can extend into the neck giving the plunging ranula, and when it is due to partial obstruction of ducts, proximal portion dilate giving a frog-belly consistency in the floor of the mouth; retention phenomenon.

Diagnosis should be provisionally made based on the physical findings and history. If the swelling has resorbed bone considerably clinical examinations may reveal "egg-shell crackling" and consistency result. Complete resorption of bone produces fluctuancy.

Following provisional diagnosis, radiological examination and few other investigations may be necessary to confirm the diagnosis.

DIAGNOSTIC INVESTIGATIONS

1. Needle Aspiration biopsy, presence and identification of cholesterol clefts, hyaline/Rushton bodies in some cysts, estimation of proteins (ratio of albumins and globulins, presence of cytokeratins, in the cystic fluid, cytology smear from the aspirated fluid.
2. Periapical radiographs are needed to determine relationship to the roots.
3. Orthopanthomogram may be necessary to confirm the diagnosis and extent of the swellings. When this panoramic view is not available, posterior-anterior view of the skull with oblique lateral for the mandible and occipito-mental view of the skull with true lateral of the skull for the upper jaw are useful.
4. Helical CT scan may be necessary to see posterior and basal skull extensions of the cyst
5. 3D Ultrasound imaging is very useful, reliable and cheaper for diagnoses of soft tissue cysts.
6. Magnetic resonance imaging scan with both T1 and T2 weighted images will be useful for large, extensive soft tissue cysts like cystic hygroma.
7. Incisional and excisional biopsies should be done based on the type and extent of the lesion.

8. Immunocytochemistry or immunohistochemitry to detect ground substances, mucins, hyaline bodies, calcifications, cytokeratins, vimentins, matrix metalloproteins, and so on.

Goals in the Management of Cysts

1. Decompression of the intra-cystic pressure.
2. Eliminating their cyst lining.
3. Preservation of teeth if possible.
4. Preservation of neighboring vital anatomic structures.
5. Prevention of recurrence of the cyst.

Operative Procedures for Management of Cysts

Depending on the type, size and nature of cyst, treatment can be

- Enucleation of cyst with primary closure
- Enucleation of cyst with peripheral ostectomy, chemical cauterization and primary closure
- Enucleation of the cyst with packaging and delayed closure
- Enucleation with primary closure and bone grafting

Marsupialization of cyst-opening the cyst to allow continuity and replacement of cystic lining, with the oral mucosa which releases fibroblastic and epithelial growth factors for healing, remodeling and granulation tissue formation from the base of the cavity and normal epithelial regeneration.

Cyst lining must always be sent for histopathological examination. Our experience has shown that most of the initial histological diagnoses of cysts obtained from small tissues taken during incision biopsies are not very dependable and misleading to the surgeons as some of these lesions eventually turn out to be unicystic ameloblastoma after histological processing of post-operative specimens.

Therefore, when marsupialization is done for large cysts, apart from the fact that diagnosis must be certain, close monitoring, serial extraoral radiographs and regular follow up must be emphasized to the patient.

Evaluation and Management of Specific Cysts

True Cyst or Epithelial Cysts

Developmental Odontogenic Cyst

Dentigerous Cyst

- Also called follicular cyst.
- Separation of the follicle from around the crown of an unerupted or partially erupted tooth leads to its origin.
- It covers the crown of the tooth and is attached to enamel junction.
- Developmental cyst and its tissue of origin is reduced enamel epithelium.
- Fluid accumulation due to obstruction between the reduced enamel epithelium and crown of an interrupted tooth leads to the formation of the dentigerous cysts.

Clinical Features

- Mostly in the age range of 10 -30 yrs
- More common in males
- More common in mandible.
- It mostly involves interrupted mandibular third molars, though other sites such as maxillary canines, maxillary third molars and mandibular second premolars are also involved.
- On examining clinically it reveals a missing tooth or teeth and mostly a hard swelling which results in facial asymmetry
- It is asymptomatic, occasionally patient presents with pain or swelling

Central Type Dentigerous Cyst
Most common and it surround the crown of the tooth and the crown projects into the cyst

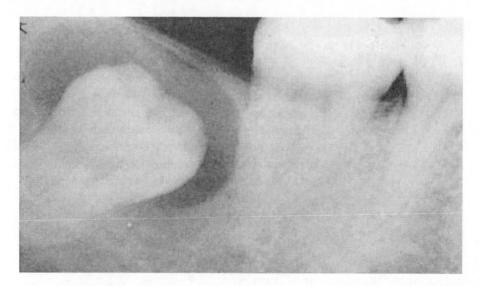

Figure 1. Periapical radiograph showing central type of dentigerous cyst around lower third molar.

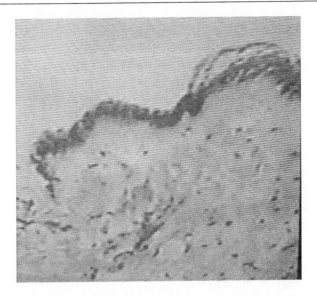

Figure 2. Photomicrograph showing dentigerous cyst lined with non-keratinized stratified squamous epithelium.

Circumferential Dentigerous Cyst

Surrounds the entire crown but does not involve the occlusal surface, so the tooth may erupt through the cyst.

The Lateral Dentigerous Cyst

Usually associated with mesioangular impacted mandibular third molars where the cyst grows laterally along the root surface and only partially surrounds the crown

Radiographic Features

It presents a well circumscribed unilocular radiolucency around crown of tooth.

Histology

Epithelium is non keratinized stratified squamous epithelium, about 4-6 cells thick. It has a fibrous connective tissue wall, with areas of chronic inflammation, hyalinization and calcifications.

Differential Diagnosis

- Odontogenic kerotocyst
- Unicystic ameloblastoma
- Calcifying epithelial odontogenic tumor (Pindborg tumor)
- Adenomatoid odontogenic tumor
- Eruption cyst

Management

- Treated by surgical removal, which usually involves the tooth as well.

- Large cysts may be treated by marsupialization.
- The cyst lining should be sent for histologic examination because ameloblastomas have been reported to occur in the cyst lining.

Eruption Cyst

- Also called eruption hematoma.
- Develops as a result of separation of dental follicle from around the crown of an erupting tooth
- It is a developmental cyst.
- Tissue of origin is reduced enamel epithelium

Clinical Features

- Mostly in children less than 10 yrs age.
- Seen as soft translucent swelling in the gingival mucosa overlying the crown of an erupting deciduous or permanent teeth
- Any erupting tooth, 1st permanent molars and maxillary incisors are most frequently involved.
- Blue to dark red in color due to presence of blood in the cystic fluid

Treatment

- No treatment is required as the cyst often ruptures spontaneously permitting the tooth to erupt
- Surgically exposing the crown of the tooth helps in tooth eruption.

Odontogenic Keratocyst (OKC)

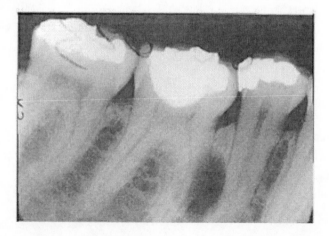

Figure 3. Periapical radiograph showing odontogenic keratocyst around lower molars.

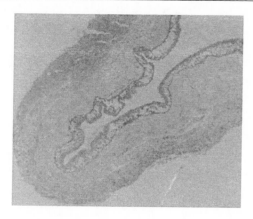

Figure 4. Photomicrograph showing odontogenic keratocyst with convoluted parakeratinized stratified squamous epithelium with a prominent basal layer.

- Derived from the remnants of the dental lamina, with production of p53 protein, accumulation of squames and keratin materials, interleukin release, pressure bone resorption and intrabony expansion.
- High recurrence rate.
- It is a developmental cyst.
- Tissue of origin is dental lamina
- Epithelium appears to have innate growth potential, lined by thin stratified squamous epithelium, about 8-10 cells thick, parakeratinized type constitute about 70%, orthokeratinized, 15% and mixed about 15%, tomb-stone arrangement of basal cells which make them prominent, fibrous connective tissue, with areas of chronic inflammation, multiple budding and penetration of daughter cells into cortical bone.
- Wide age range from infancy to old age
- Commonly present as intrabony mass and more in males
- 70-80% cases involve the mandible / ascending ramus
- Asymptomatic unless secondarily infected
- Enlarges in antero-posterior direction without causing gross bony expansion, swelling is minimal, but when left untreated for long it can produce buccolingual expansion, as more bone is resorbed, consistency changes from bony hard to ping-pong/tennis ball to egg-shell and finally fluctuant when all the bone overlying the capsule is resorbed.
- Aspiration reveals a thick, yellow, cheesy material (keratin).
- An aspirate of less than 4.0 gm of soluble protein level is indicative of OKC.

Primordial cysts originate from the stellate reticulum and have prominent rete pegs but other features are similar to OKC.

Gorlin- Gortz Syndrome

Multiple odontogenic keratocyst swellings occur in different sites of the jaw bones in Gorlin-Gortz syndrome, it is commoner in children and present with dental anarchy and other features like:

- Desmoid tumors of the skin
- Basal cell carcinomas
- Naevoid cell tumors
- Hyperparathyroidism and other pituitary gland endocrine tumors may be found, with mild hypercalcemia and hypophosphatasia
- Bifid ribs
- Multiple nodules on clavicle, ribs, sternum, vertebrae
- Pathologic fractures, dystrophic/metastatic calcification
- Calcification of the falx cerebri
- Hyperpigmentations

Radiographic Features

- Well demarcated unilocular or multilocular radiolucency with a scalloped, radiopaque margin
- May be associated with interrupted tooth.

Differential Diagnosis

- dentigerous cyst
- ameloblastoma
- odontogenic myxoma
- adenomatoid odontogenic tumor
- ameloblastic fibroma

Treatment of Odontogenic Keratocyst and Primordial Cyst

Conservative Surgery
Enucleation, peripheral ostectomy with vulcanite bur and chemical curettage with Carnoy's solution (95% absolute alcohol, glacial acetic acid, ferric chloride and chloroform)

Radical Surgery
When lesion is large, longstanding, perforation and invasion into soft tissues, high reccurence rate and considering the fact some authors now believe that it is a tumor especially the parakeratinized type with p53 protein identification, it is better to do resection and reconstruction of the affected jaw.

Glandular Odontogenic Cyst

- Glandular odontogenic cyst
- It is a rare odontogenic cyst
- It is also known as sialo-odontogenic cyst because of its histological features.
- It is commoner in the mandible than maxilla.

- It has equal sex predilection and the mean age of occurrence is 50 years but it has a wide range from second to the ninth decade.
- Most cases present multilocular radioluscency
- This cyst is lined by nonkeratinized epithelium containing ciliated columnar cells. Mucous cells containing mucin are found within the epithelium.

Treatment

- Surgical excision

Long term follow-up is necessary because of its potential to reoccur.

Gingival Cyst of Infants
Also known as

- Gingival Cyst of Newborn
- Dental lamina Cyst of Newborn
- Epstein Pearls
- Bohn's Nodules

Cinical Features

- More common in new born infants
- Small, single or multiple keratin-filled cysts on the alveolus.
- Epstein's pearls- Along the midpalatine raphae, small keratin filled cysts/ nodules found probably derived from the entrapped epithelial remnants along the line of fusion.
- Bohn's Nodules- Small keratin-filled cysts/nodules scattered over the palate, mostly along the junction of hard and soft palate and derived from the salivary gland structures.

Pathogenesis

- arises from dental lamina
- Epithelial remnants of dental lamina have the capacity to proliferate, keratinize and form small cysts
- Parakeratinized stratified squamous epithelium and keratin fills the cyst cavity.
- Because of pressure from the cyst the overlying oral epithelium may be atrophic.

Treatment
They atrophy and disappear once the contents are expelled.

Inflammatory Odontogenic Cyst

Radicular Cyst

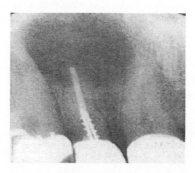

Figure 5. Periapical radiograph showing radicular cyst around the root filled non-vital upper left lateral incisors.

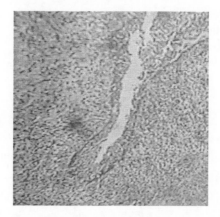

Figure 6. Photomicrograph showing radicular cyst lined non-keratinized squamous epithelium with numerous chronic inflammatory cells within the epithelium and connective tissue wall.

- Also known as apical periodontal cyst, periapical cyst or root end cyst
- Epithelial lining is derived from epithelial rests of Malassez

A radicular cyst presupposes physical, chemical or bacterial injury resulting in death of pulp followed by stimulation of epithelial cell rests of Malaseez which are present normally in periodontal ligament.

Pathogenesis of radicular cyst is conveniently considered in 3 phases:

1) Phase of Initiation,
2) Phase of cyst formation,
3) Phase of cyst Enlargement

1) Phase of Initiation: It is generally agreed that the epithelial lining of these cysts are derived from epithelial cell rests of Malassez in periodontal ligaments. However in some cases, epithelial lining may be derived from:

a) Respiratory epithelium of maxillary sinus when periapical lesion communicates with sinus wall.
b) Oral epithelium from fistulous tract.
c) Oral epithelium proliferating apically from periodontal pocket.

The mechanism of stimulation of epithelial cells to proliferate is not clear. It may be due to inflammation in periapical granuloma or some products of dead pulp may initiate the process at the same time it evokes an inflammatory reaction.

In addition, there is evidence of local changes in supporting connective tissue which may be responsible for activating the cell rests of Malassez. Reduced oxygen tension, high carbon-dioxide level and increased acidity (low pH) within the periapical tissues.

2) Phase of cyst formation: It is a process by which cavity becomes lined by proliferating epithelium.

There are two proposed theories-

a) Most widely accepted theory suggests that initial reaction leading to cyst formation is a proliferation of epithelial rests in periapical area involved by granuloma. As the proliferation continue with the epithelial mass increasing in size by division of the cells on periphery corresponding to basal layer of surface epithelium. The cells of central portion of mass become separated away from oxygen and nutrition in comparison with basal layer, degeneration and liquefactive necrosis occur. This creates an epithelium lined cavity filled with fluid.
b) The second theory states that a cyst may form through proliferation of epithelium to line a pre-existing cavity formed through focal necrosis and degeneration of connective tissue in periapical granuloma. But the finding of epithelium or epithelial proliferation near an area of necrosis is not common.

3) Phase of cyst enlargement: Experimental work provided evidence that osmosis makes contribution to increase in size of cyst. Investigators found that fluids of radicular cysts have Gamma Globulin level High by almost more than half to patient's own serum. Plasma protein exudate and hyaluronic acid as well as products of cell breakdown contribute to high osmotic pressure of cystic fluid on cyst walls which causes resorption of bone & enlargement of cyst.

Microbiology
Cyst may or may not be infected. Whenever infection is present Actinomyces organisms have been isolated from radicular cyst commonly.

Microorganisms mainly found in root canal are 75% Gram positive and 25% Gram negative, among which Streptococci are predominant' also other Gram positive organisms like Staphylococci, Cornybacterium, yeast and others are found. Gram negative organisms are Spirochetes, Nesseria, Bacteroids, fusobacterium, pseudomonas etc. In periapical lesions like radicular cysts, obligate anaerobes are found. In long-standing cases of periapical pathology alpha hemolytic and non hemolytic streptococci also constitute flora.

Medias used for Culture

- Brain Heart Infusion Broath with 0.1% Agar
- Trylicase Soy Broath with 0.1% Agar (TSA)
- Glucose Ascitis Broath

Pathogenesis

- Initially there occurs proliferation of epithelial rests in the periapical area
- It continues with epithelial mass increasing in size by division of cells on the periphery
- The cells in the central portion become separated further away from their source of nutrition which eventually degenerate become necrotic and liquefy. This forms an epithelium lined cavity filled with fluid.

Expansion of the cyst causes erosion of the floor of the maxillary sinus. As soon as it enters the maxillary antrum the expansion starts to occur a little faster because there is space available for expansion. Tapping the affected teeth will cause pain. This is virtually diagnostic of pulpal infection.

Clinical Features

A) Frequency: It is most common cystic lesion of jaw comprising about approximately 52.3% of jaw cystic lesions
B) Age: Many cases are found in 4th & 5th decades of life after which there is gradual decline.
C) Sex: It is more common in males comprising about 58% and in females comprising 42%.
D) Race: Caucasians are affected about twice than blacks.
E) Site: It occurs with frequency of 60% in Maxilla. Though it may occur in all tooth bearing areas of both the jaws but preferably it occurs in maxillary anterior region. Upper lateral Incisors and 'Dens in Dente' are usually the offending teeth. It occurs most commonly at apices of involved teeth. They may however be found at lateral accessory root canals.

Clinical Presentation

Smaller radicular cysts are usually symptomless and are found in relation with non-vital teeth when periapical x-rays are taken.

Larger lesions show slowly enlarging swelling. At first the enlargement is bony hard but as cyst increases in size, the covering bone becomes very thin, despite subperiosteal deposition & swelling exhibits springiness, only when bone has become completely eroded, the bone will show fluctuation.

In maxilla, there may be buccal and palatal enlargement but in mandible it is usually labial or buccal and rarely lingual. But for upper lateral incisors, it is palatal because of the palatal orientation of the roots.

Features include pain when infected. These cysts are usually painless unless infected. However, complain of pain may be observed in patient without any evidence of infection when there is pressure on the nerves.

Occasionally, a discharging sinus may lead from cyst cavity to the oral mucosa. Quite often there may be more than one radicular cyst. Scientists believe that there are cyst prone individuals who show particular susceptibility to develop radicular cysts.

Radicular cysts arising from deciduous tooth are very rare. Deciduous tooth which has been treated endodontically with materials containing formecresol which in combination with tissue protein is antigenic and may elicit a humoral or cell-mediated response like rapid buccal expansion of cyst.

On rare occasion, there may be occurrence of parasthesia or there may be pathologic fracture of jaw bone take place.

Radiographically it is difficult to differentiate granuloma from a cyst. If the lesion is large, it is more likely to be a cyst. Both granuloma and cyst appear radiolucent, associated with the apex of non vital tooth.

Radiographic Features: Intra-oral periapical radiographs are useful for diagnosis. Radicular cysts are round or ovoid radiolucent areas surrounded by a narrow radio-opaque margin, which extends from lamina dura of involved tooth. In infected or rapidly enlarging cysts, radio-opaque margins may not be seen. Root resorption is rare but may occur.

Other features of radicular cyst seen on radiograph are -

Periphery and Shape- Periphery usually have a well defined cortical border. If cyst is secondarily infected, the inflammatory reaction of surrounding bone may result in loss of this cortex or alteration of cortex into more sclerotic border. The outline of radicular cyst usually is curved or circular unless it is influenced by surrounding structures such as cortical boundaries.

Internal structure- In most cases, internal structure of radicular cyst is radiolucent. Occasionally, dystrophic calcification may develop in long standing cysts appearing as sparsely distributed, small particulate radio-opacities.

Effects on surrounding structures- If a radicular cyst is large, displacement and resorption of roots of adjacent teeth may occur. The resorption pattern may have a curved outline. In rare cases, the cyst may resorb the roots of related non-vital teeth. The cyst may invaginate the antrum, but there should be evidence of a cortical boundary between contents of cyst and internal structure of antrum. The outer cortical plates of maxilla and mandible may expand in a curved or circular shape. Cyst may displace the mandibular alveolar nerve canal in an inferior direction.

Gross Features

Gross Specimen may be spheroidal or ovoid intact cystic masses, but often they are irregular and collapsed. The walls vary from extremely thin to a thickness of about 5mm. The inner surface may be smooth or corrugated yellow mural nodules of cholesterol may project into the cavity. The fluid contents are usually brown from breakdown of blood and when cholesterol crystals are present they impart a shimmering gold or straw color.

Histopathological Features: The gross specimen may be spherical or ovoid intact cystic masses, but often they are irregular and collapsed. The walls vary from extremely thin to a thickness of about 5mm. The inner surface may be smooth or corrugated. The histopathological studies shows following features –

1) Epithelial Lining: Almost all radicular cysts are wholly or in part lined by stratified squamous epithelium and thickness ranges from 1 to 50 cell layers. The only exception to this is in those rare cases of periapical lesions of maxillary sinus. In such cases, cyst is then lined with a pseudo stratified ciliated columnar epithelium or respiratory type of epithelium. Secretory cells or ciliated cells are frequently found in epithelial lining.

2) Rushton's Hyaline Bodies: In about 10% of cases of radicular cysts, Rushton's hyaline bodies are found in the epithelial linings. Very rarely they are found in the fibrous capsule. The hyaline bodies are tiny linear or arc shaped bodies which are amorphous in structure, eosinophillic in reaction and brittle in nature.

3) Cholesterol Clefts: Deposition of cholesterol crystals are found in many radicular cysts, slow but considerable amount of cholesterol accumulation could occur through degeneration and disintegration of lymphocytes, plasma cells and macrophages taking part in inflammatory process, with consequent release of cholesterol from their walls.

4) Fibrous Capsule: Fibrous capsule of radicular cyst is composed of mainly condensed parallel bundles of collagen fibres peripherally and a loose connective tissue adjacent to epithelial lining.

5) Inflammatory Cells: Acute inflammatory cells are present when epithelium is proliferating. Chronic inflammatory cells are present in connective tissue immediately adjacent to epithelium.

6) Mast cells, remnants of odontogenic epithelium and occasionally satellite microcysts are also present. Some cysts are vascularized and calcifications are also present.

Treatment of Radicular Cyst

Enucleation, root end resection and retrograde root filling.

Developmental/Inflammatory Odontogenic Cyst

Lateral Periodontal Cyst

In the younger patients, it occurs on the lateral surface of the roots as a developmental lesion, which can even be multiple giving the Butyroides' appearance on periapical x-ray.

In the much older patients it can occur following inflammation from lateral/accessory canal, low grade or incompletely treated periodontal abscess or rarely perio-endodontic lesion with inflammation extending from the apical root canal to the lateral surface of the roots.

More rarely, an established radicular (periapical) cyst extending to the lateral surface of the roots or a lateral dentigerous cyst may extend to the lateral surface of the root mimicking a lateral periodontal cyst.

Usually, the developmental lateral periodontal cyst is a co-incidental finding on x-ray presenting with small unilocular or multiple grape-like radiolucencies with no pain and no loss of vitality, but when the tooth associated is non vital, it is inflammatory in origin.

Non-odontogenic Cysts

Nasolabial Cyst

- Derived from remnants of the inferior portion of the nasolacrimal duct.
- It may arise from the epithelial rests at fusion lines of the globular portion of the medial nasal, lateral nasal, and maxillary processes or from the nasolacrimal duct
- Asymptomatic. Slowly enlarging soft tissue swelling obliterates the nasolabial fold
- Occurs in the region of the maxillary lip and base of ala, lateral to the midline
- are less than 1.5 cm
- Age ranges from 12 to 75 years, with a mean age of 44 years.
- Mostly in females.

Radiographic Features

- Soft tissue lesion located adjacent to the alveolar process above the incisors apices.
- Being a soft tissue lesion, plain radiographs may not show any changes.
- The investigation could include computed tomography (CT) or magnetic resonance imaging (MRI)

Differential Diagnosis

- The swelling caused by an infected nasolabial cyst may mimick an acute dentoalveolar abscess or
- Nasal furuncle, if it pushes upward into the floor of the nasal cavity or
- Mucous extravasation cyst or a cystic salivary adenoma

Treatment
Surgical excision

Nasopalatine Duct Cyst

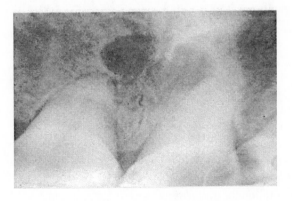

Figure 7. Periapical radiograph showing nasopalatine cyst.

- Also called as Incisive canal cyst;
- Commonest of non-odontogenic cyst
- Derived from epithelial remnants of naso-palatine duct

Clinical Features

- May develop at any age but most common in 4 – 6 decades
- Slow growing swelling with occasional salty taste discharge.
- Large cyst may cause mid palatine swelling
- Male: female ratio; 3:1.

Radiographic Features

- Radiolucent area with well defined margins.
- Heart shaped radiolucency and septate trifurcation within it, reflecting union of the premaxilla and both maxillae
- Symmetrical about the mid line and sometimes shifted to one side

Differential Diagnosis

- Periapical granuloma
- Radicular cyst

Management

- Enucleation, preferably from the palate to avoid nasopalatine nerve.
- If cyst is large then do marsupialization.

Median Palatal Cyst

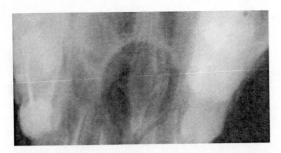

Figure 8. Occlusal radiograph showing median palatal cyst.

- Rare cyst develops from epithelium entrapped along the line of fusion of lateral palatal shelves of maxilla
- Occurs in the midline of posterior palate

- Presents as a firm or fluctuant swelling of the midline of hard palate posterior to the palatine papilla
- Occurs in young adults
- Asymptomatic
- Shows well circumscribed radioluscency in the midline of the hard palate
- Midline radioluscency without clinical evidence of expansion is probably a nasopalatine duct cyst

Treatment

- Surgical removal

Pseudocysts or Non-epithelial Cysts

Solitary Bone Cyst

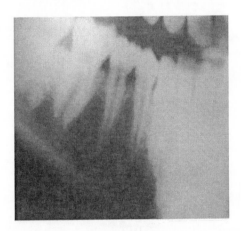

Figure 9. Periapical radiograph showing radiolucent area with traumatic bone cyst above the inferior alveolar canal lower, also destroying the interradicular bone around the lower premolars and molars.

- Also known as simple, traumatic, hemorrhagic, and unicameral cyst
- Usually related to trauma
- Represent hemodynamic disturbances in medullary bone

Clinical Features

- Most common in long bones and rare in jaws.
- In children and adolescents
- Involves 2-3rd decades.
- Mostly in males.
- Premolar and molar region in the mandible.
- Mostly asymptomatic

Radiographic Features

- Radiolucency usually above the inferior alveolar canal due to destruction of alveolar bone
- Regular outline common, prominent around and between the standing teeth
- Well defined margin

Management

- Curettage

Aneurysmal Bone Cyst

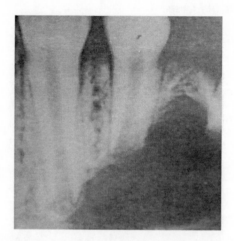

Figure 10. Periapical radiograph showing radiolucent area caused by aneurysmal bone cyst below the open apices of the lower canine and premolar.

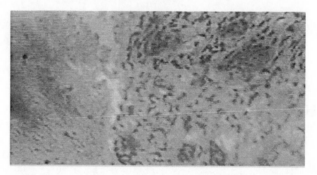

Figure 11. Photomicrogragh of aneurysmal bone cyst showing numerous multinucleated giant cells within the fibrous connective tissue and a blood filled space to the left.

The cyst arises from venous malformations within the medullary system due to venous obstruction with intravenous pressure, increased vascular sinusoids, fibrocellular proliferation and bony expansion; may be associated with trauma or bone disease like central giant cell granuloma and fibrous dysplasia.

- Rare cyst of the jaws, benign, rapidly growing osteolytic lesion, characterized by blood filled cystic spaces lined by bony or fibrous septa
- Arise as primary lesion or secondary to bone disease
- Occurs in people less than 20 years, usually childhood
- Posterior ramus region of the mandible commonly affected
- Firm expansile swelling on bimanual palpation and causes facial deformity

Radiograph

- Uni or multilocular with ballooned out appearance due to cortical plate expansion

Histology

It presents fibrous connective tissue with variable numbers of multinucleated giant cells. Commonly seen within the connective tissue are sinusoidal spaces lined with fibroblasts and macrophages.

Management

- Surgical curettage

Gross appearance like blood soaked sponge and central hemangioma is a differential.

Stafne's Idiopathic Cyst

- Uncommon developmental anomaly of the mandible with salivary gland inclusion.
- Appears as round or oval well demarcated radiolucency between the premolar region and the angle of the jaw beneath the inferior dental canal
- Depression or concavity on the lingual aspect of the mandible
- Histology shows ectopic or aberrant salivary gland tissue within the lesion.

Soft Tissue Cysts of the Oral Cavity/Head and Neck

Majority are developmental while few are traumatic and inflammatory in origin.

Salivary Mucoceles

- Mucous extravasations cyst
- Mucous retention cyst

Mucous Extravasation Cyst

- Found In lower lip, cheek and floor of mouth and; in any age group but commonly
- Young adults
- Presents clinically as a bluish or translucent submucosa swelling
- Traumatic rupture of minor or major salivary gland duct
- Cystic space lined with compressed connective tissue and chronic inflammatory cells

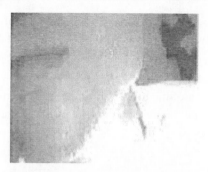

Figure 12. Preoperative photograph showing sialocele due to rupture of parotid duct.

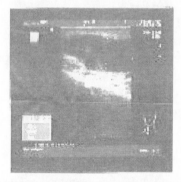

Figure 13. Showing preoperative ultrasound of the patient with sialocele from rupture of parotid duct.

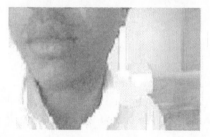

Figure 14. Post-operative photograph showing complete regression of the swelling.

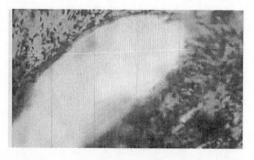

Figure 15. Photomicrograph of a mucous extravasation cyst showing the cystic cavity surrounded by compressed connective tissue and chronic inflammatory cells.

Mucous Retention Cyst

- Almost never found in the lower lip
- Derived from cystic dilatation of a duct due to obstruction and lined by ductal epithelium
- No surrounding chronic inflammatory reaction

Ranula

- Describes a swelling in floor of mouth which resemble a frog's belly
- Most ranulas are mucous extravasation cysts
- Ranula may extend through the mylohyoid muscle and present in the submandibular area or neck (plunging ranula). Plunging ranula may be congenital, occurring from trapped, ectopic or aberrant minor salivary gland which duct fails to open into the mucosa.
- Treatment for plunging ranula is marsupialization and excision of the affected salivary glan

Thyroglossal Cyst

- It is derived from the residues of the embryonic thyroglossal duct. The residues usually get entrapped in the region of the hyoid bone where it can give rise to the cyst.
- Thyroid glands descend from foramen caecum of the tongue. Persistence of the duct cause fluid accumulation and enlargement forming a cyst in the midline of the neck anteriorly. The cyst moves on swallowing and on protrusion of the tongue. Thyroid gland only moves on swallowing.
- Very rarely, located in floor of the mouth and the tongue, when infected, a discharging sinus may form
- Lined by stratified squamous epithelium and thyroid follicles may be found in the wall of the cyst.

Treatment
Surgery- Cystrong's operation involve excision of the cyst, duct and midportion of the hyoid bone which can harbour the cystic duct in between.

- Ectopic thyroid gland (on the tongue) may be functioning and must not be removed until the thyroid gland in the neck is confirmed to be present and functioning normally. However, if not removed regular observation must be done to detect any transformation early.

Dermoid and Epidermoid Cysts and Cystic Teratoma
Occurs at variable sites in the head and neck including, floor of mouth and ovary
Arise from entrapment of pluripotential epithelial cells in the midline because of deranged fusion of first (mandibular) and second (hyoid) branchial arches.

Present as intra-oral or submental swellings. It is slow growing soft tissue swelling in the young adults. Extraorally, it may give a double-chin appearance when it is located below the mylohyoid muscle.

It is lined by a layer of orthokeratinized stratified squamous epithelium when the origin is ectodermal while those with endodermal origin, the epithelium is pseudostratified columnar with cilia and goblet cells. The lumen contains keratin. Skin appendages like hair follicles, sweat glands and sebaceous glands are present in the cystic wall of dermoid cyst but absent in the wall of epidermoid cyst. Cystic teratomas may also contain additional structures such as nerve, teeth and bone.

Treatment

Excision

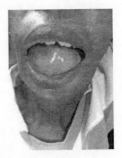

Figsure 16. Photographs showing dermoid cyst in a 32yr-old male patient that caused airway obstruction.

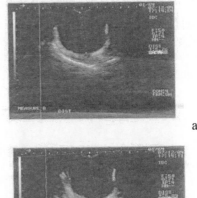

a

b

Figure 17 a and b. Pre-operative ultrasound images of the 32yr-old showing grossly enlarged tongue measuring 5.76cm by 6.38cm with a huge moderately demarcated cystic space of dimensions 5.76cm by 6.3cm containing sedimented, mixed echogenic debris. The normal fibrillar echopattern of the extrinsic muscles was intact while that for the intrinsic muscles was lost.

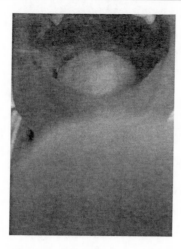

Figure 18. Three weeks post operative photograph of the 32yr-old, tongue has remarkably reduced in size.

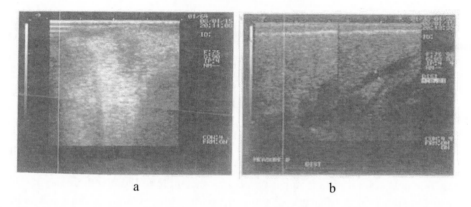

a   b

Figure 19 a and b. Post- operative ultrasound of the dermoid cyst in the 32yr-old showed the size of the tongue had reduced to 2.1cm by 2.24cm.The intrinsic muscles showed better fibrillation though still echogenic, the cystic space had resolved and was now possible to distinguish between the anterior serous and distal mucous regions of the dorsum of the tongue.

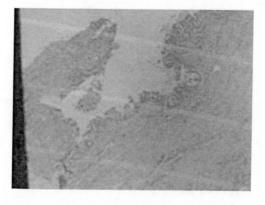

Figure 20. Photomicrograph of the dermoid cystic lesion in the 32yr-old lined with pseudo- stratified columnar epithelium. No skin appendages are seen within the cystic wall. Magnification × 10.

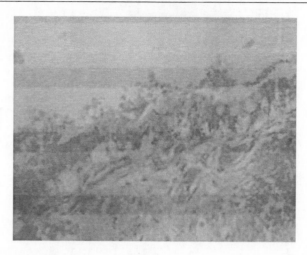

Figure 21. Photomicrograph showing areas of pseudo-stratified columnar epithelium with Goblet's cells in the cystic lining. Magnification × 40.

Cystic Hygroma

Cystic hygroma is a large fluctuant mass found in the neck of the newly born; may often obstruct or prolong labor; shows the same histologic appearance as cavernous lymphangioma with multiple lymphatic sinuses.

Treatment

Excision

Branchial/Lymphoepithelial Cyst

Branchial cyst is found in the upper part below the angle of the mandible in young adults; remnants of branchial cleft (pharyngeal groove) between the second and third arches lined by stratified squamous epithelium, its wall contains organized lymphoid tissues.

Treatment

Excision

Complications of Cyst

1. Secondary Infection: Cyst may get secondarily infected and infection can spread.
2. Pathologic Jaw Fracture: Cyst can erode the bone particularly when it is present in posterior region and it may cause pathologic jaw bone fracture.
3. Carcinomatous/Neoplastic Changes: Squamous cell carcinoma or epidermoid carcinoma may occasionally arise from epithelial lining of a cyst. Odontogenic tumour like Ameloblastoma has been reported to arise from the wall of some odontogenic cyst, particularly dentigerous cyst.
4. Cystic hygroma may obstruct labor

REFERENCES

Bailey, et al. In Head & Neck Surgery – Otolaryngology. Eds. Dierks, E and Bernstein, M. *Odontogenic cysts, tumors, and related jaw lesions.* 2nd edition. Volume 2(108): 1541-1562.

Bataineh, A, Al Qudah, M. Treatment of mandibular odontogenic keratocysts. *Oral Surg Oral Med Oral Pathol Oral Radiol Endod.* 1998; 86(1): 42-47.

Bialek EJ, Jakubowski W, Zajkowski P, Szopinsk. K, Osmolski A. Ultrasound of the major salivary glands: Anatomy and spatial relationships, pathologic conditions and pitfalls. *RadioGraphics* 2006; 26:745-763.

Blotta P, Pastore A, Tugnoli V, Galatis LT., Parnes SM. Management of parotid sialocele with botulinium toxin. *Laryngoscope* 1999; 109: 1344-1346.

Brusati R, Galiotos S, Tullio A, Moscato G. The midline saggital glossotomy for treatment of dermoid cyst of the floor of the mouth. *J Oral Maxillofac Surg* 1991; 49: 875-878.

Cant PJ, Campbell JA. Management of traumatic parotid sialoceles and fistulae: a prospective study. *Aust NZJ Surg* 1991; 61(10): 742-743.

Chow TL, Kwok SP. Use of botulinium toxin type A in a case of parotid sialocele. *Hong kong Med J* 2003; 9: 293-294.

DelBalso AM (1995). "Lesions of the jaws". Semin. *Ultrasound CT MR* 1974; 16 (6): 487–512

Devine JC, Jones DC. Carcinomatous transformation of sublingual dermoid cyst. A case report. *Int J Oral Maxillofac Surg.* 2000; 29: 126-127.

Dimov Zh, Dimov K, Kr'stev N, Kr'stev D, Baeva N, Baeva M, Yar'mov N. Dermoid, epidermoid and teratoid cyst of the tongue and oral cavity floor. *Khirurgiia.* (Sofiia). 2000; 56: 30-32.

Kahn, Michael A. *Basic Oral and Maxillofacial Pathology.* Volume 1. 2001.

Koeller KK, Alamo L. Adair CF, Smirniotopoulos JG. Congental cystic masses of the neck: Radiologic and Pathologic correlation. *Radiographics.* 1999; 19: 121-146.

Koppang, H, et al. Glandular odontogenic cyst: report of two cases and literature review of 45 previously reported cases. *J Oral Pathol Med.* 1998; 27(9): 455-462.

Lohaus M, Hansmann J, Witzel A, Flectenmatcher C, Mende U, Reisser C. Uncommon sonographic findings of epidermoid cyst in the head and neck. *HNO* 1999; 47: 737-740.

Lapid O, Kreiger Y, Sagi A. Use of transdermal scopolamine, Scopoderm TTS. *Aesthetic Plastic Surgery* 2004; 28: 24-28.

Miles LP, Naidoo LC, Reddy J. Congenital dermoid cyst of the tongue. *J laryngol Otol* 1997; 111: 1179-82.

Mrad DK, Zriq A, Mhiri-souri M, Arifa- Achour N, Khochtali H, Tlili-Graies K. Intra-lingual dermoid cyst. *J Radiol* 2005; 86: 502-505.

Myssiorek D, Lee J, Wasserman P, Lustrin E. Intralingual dermoid cyst. A report of 2 new cases. *Ear Nose Throat J* 2000; 79: 380-383.

Obiechina AE, Arotiba JT, Ogunbiyi JO. Coexisting congenital sublingual dermoid and bronchogenic cyst. *Br J Oral Maxillofac Surg* 1999; 37: 58-60.

Pancholi A, Sameer R, Prakash AV, Vijay Vaidya. Midline epidermoid cyst: A rare case. *The Internet Journal of Otorhinolaryngology.* 2006; 4.

Parekh D, Glezerson G, Stewart M, Esver J, Lawson HH. Post-traumatic parotid fistulae and sialoceles. A prospective study of conservative management of 51 cases. *Ann Surg* 1989; 209: 105-111.

Ramer, M, Mantazem, A, Lane, S, Lumerman, H. Glandular odontogenic cyst: Report of a case and review of the literature. *Oral Surg Oral Med Oral Pathol Oral Radiol Endod.* 1997; 84(1): 54-57.

Rushton VE, Pemberton MN. Salivary Otorrhoea: A case report and a review of the literature. *Dentomaxillofacial Radiology* 2005; 34:376-379.

Sela J, Ulmansky M. Mucous retention cyst of salivary glands. *J Oral Surg* 1969; 27(8): 619-623.

Shaari CM, Ho BT, Shah K, Biller HF. Lingual dermoid cyst. *Otorlaryngol Head and Neck Surg* 1995; 112: 476-478.

Smirniotopoulos J, Chiechi M. Teratomas, dermoids, and epidermoids of the head and neck. *RadioGraphics* 1995; 15: 1437-1455.

Solomon AR, Mcclatchey KD, Batsakis JG. Serous extravasation granuloma. A parotid mass. *Arch Otolaryngol* 1981; 107(5): 294-296.

Toida, M. So-called calcifying odontogenic cyst: review and discussion on the terminology and classification. *J Oral Pathol Med.* 27(2): 49-52. 1998.

Vogl T, Steger W, Ihrier S, Ferrara P, Grevers G. Cystic masses in the floor of the mouth. Value of MR imaging in planning surgery. *AJR* 1993; 161: 183-186.

Zeltser R, Milhem I, Azaz B. Hasson O. Dermoid cysts of the floor of the mouth. A report of four cases. *Am J Otorlarygol.* 2000; 21: 55-60.

In: Cysts: Causes, Diagnosis and Treatment Options   ISBN: 978-1-62081-315-7
Editors: A. Mendes Ortiz and A. Jimenez Moreno   © 2012 Nova Science Publishers, Inc.

Chapter 7

THE MALIGNANT POTENTIAL OF EPIDERMAL AND VERRUCOUS CUTANEOUS CYSTS

Teresa Pusiol[1]*, Doriana Morichetti[1],†, Reinhard Kluge[2],‡
and Esther Hanspeter[2],§

[1]Institute of Pathology, Rovereto Hospital, Rovereto (TN), Italy
[2]Institute of Pathology, Bolzano Hospital, Bolzano (BZ), Italy

ABSTRACT

The malignant potential of cutaneous cysts is studied. We have examined 7 squamous cell carcinoma (SCC) arising in epidermal cyst (EC). The age at presentation ranged from 60 to 96 years. In all cases histological examination revealed a cyst lined by stratified squamous epithelium exhibiting keratinisation. The cystic epithelium showed in situ SCC squamous cell carcinoma in continuity with invasive keratinizing component. The study for HPV was negative. Perineal cystic nodule was found in a 86 year-old woman. The wall showed varying degrees of papillomatosis, hypergranulosis, parakeratosis with dysplastic and koilocytic changes. An invasive SCC squamous cell carcinoma was found in continuity with in situ malignant cystic epithelium. Using polymerase chain reaction and in situ hybridization, we have detected the presence of human papillomavirus (HPV) genotype 16 in the cystic wall and in the invasive carcinoma. CT scan showed a diffuse wall thickening of the anorectal region and infiltration of anus levators muscle. The histopathology examination of endoscopic biopsies of the anal canal and rectum revealed a SCC squamous cell carcinoma with presence of HPV 16. The patient refused any kind of treatment. The diagnosis of SCC arising from verrucous cyst (HPV associated cyst) was performed with extensive involvement of anal canal. A lesion may be diagnosed as "SCC arising in an EC" only with the support of an accurate histological documentation in order to exclude mimics (proliferating epidermoid cyst, proliferating trichilemmal cyst, and pseudocarcinomatous

---

* Address for correspondence: Teresa Pusiol , Institute of Anatomic Pathology, S. Maria del Carmine Hospital, Piazzale S. Maria 6, 38068 Rovereto (TN), Italy, E-mail: teresa.pusiol@apss.tn.it.
† E-mail: doriana.morichetti@apss.tn.it.
‡ E-mail: reinhard.kluge@asbz.it.
§ E-mail: esther.hanspeter@asbz.it.

hyperplasia in a ruptured cyst). HPV demonstration has to be negative in order to exclude a verrucous cyst. The main histological feature essential for diagnosis is the presence of a "continuum" between cystic wall and SCC. Appling this diagnostic criterion many reported cases shouldn't been classified in this group. Despite the low risk of malignant transformation, it is generally agreed that all suspected cutaneous cysts should be submitted for histological examination. Regarding verrucous cyst, the site, the malignant transformation, the finding of HPV 16 type and the extensive neoplastic involvement of adjacent organ may be considered features of an extraordinary rare case.

INTRODUCTION

Epidermal cysts (ECs) are solitary, dome shaped, freely movable, slowly growing lesions with a predilection for the trunk, neck and face. They are thought to be derived from the pilosebaceous follicle, but they may arise from implantation of the epidermis, particularly on the palms and soles and in the subungual region. The malignant transformation of EC is an very unusual finding. This very rare malignant disease is an enigmatic pathological event and it is difficult to find in human pathology a malignancy so easy to diagnose and so surprising. Cases of malignant transformation reported in the older literature have been questioned as some, at least, represent proliferating trichilemmal cysts or proliferating epidermal cysts. Verrucous cyst (VC) is a type of cutaneous cyst with microscopy features consistent with Human papilloma virus (HPV) infection. Only HPV 57 and 60 has been identified in the cystic wall to date. These HPV types are often associated with malignant disease (high – risk HPV). It is surprising that cases of SCC arising from VC *HPAC* has not been reported to date. In the present study we report seven cases of SCC arising in EC and the first case of SCC arising in perineal VC with simultaneous extensive neoplastic involvement of anal canal.

MATERIALS AND METHODS

Seven cases of SCC arising in EC and one case in perineal VC with simultaneous extensive neoplastic involvement of anal canal has been examined.

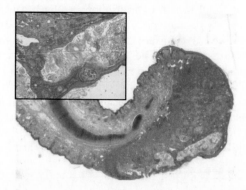

Figure 1. Squamous cell carcinoma arising in epidermal cyst of the right helix. The macroscopic illustration show cystic cutaneous lesions and helix cartilage. The cystic epithelium show acanthosis, hyperkeratosis, dysplastic change and it is in continuity with carcinomatous proliferations. (H&E *HandE*;40x) (insert).

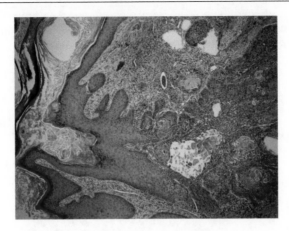

Figure 2. Squamous cell carcinoma arising in epidermal cyst. The histological section show typical epidermal cyst, lined by a stratified squamous epithelium with granular cell layer. The epithelium showed dysplastic area in continuity with carcinoma. Granulomatous inflammation is evident corresponding to cystic parietal rupture. The cystic lumen contains keratin fragments (H&E *HandE*;40x).

The medical records for each case were reviewed and the following attributes were recorded: age, sex, duration and location. The lesions were fixed in phosphate-buffered formalin and embedded in paraffin. Sections were stained with haematoxylin-eosin. Serial sections of all specimens had been prepared in order to verify that the cystic appearance was real and not merely the result of poor orientation of the specimen. In all cases sections of paraffin-embedded tissue were investigated for the presence of HPV-DNA sequences by polymerase chain reaction (PCR) and in situ hybridization.

RESULTS

Squamous Cell Carcinoma Arising in Epidermal Cyst

In all cases histopathological examination revealed a cyst lined by stratified squamous epithelium exhibiting keratinization. The cystic epithelium showed *in situ* SCC in continuity with invasive keratinizing component. PCR and in situ hybridization for HPV research were negative. A diagnosis of invasive SCC arising in the wall of an EC was performed in all cases (Figures 1 and 2).

Squamous Cell Carcinoma Arising in Verrucous Cyst

An 86-year-old woman presented with a perineal nodule 1.5cm in diameter that she had noticed for the first time about a month and a half earlier. No viral warts were seen near the lesion. The wide excision of the lesion was performed. Gross pathologic examination identified cystic tumour.The histology of the VC showed varying degrees of papillomatosis, hypergranulosis, parakeratosis and squamous eddy formation. Koilocytic changes with large keratohyaline granules were noted. Areas of cystic in situ SCC with an invasive component were found adjacent to dysplastic epithelium (Figure 3).

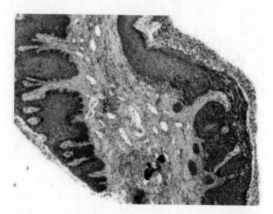

Figure 3. Squamous cell carcinoma arising in human papillomavirus associated cyst. The invasive squamous carcinomatous component in continuity is evident (H&E *HandE*; 100X).

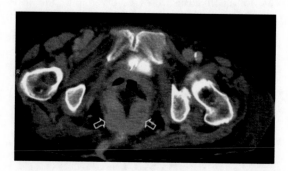

Figure 4. Squamous cell carcinoma arising in human papillomavirus associated cyst. Enhanced CT scan of the pelvis shows diffuse wall thickening of the anorectum and infiltration of anus levator's *elevator's* muscle (arrows). No enlarged pelvic lymph nodes were revealed.

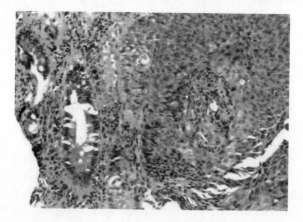

Figure 5. Infiltration by squamous cell carcinoma of the rectal mucosa is evident (H&E *HandE*; 100X).

Using polymerase chain reaction (PCR) and in situ hybridization, we have detected the presence of human papillomavirus (HPV) genotype 16 in the cystic wall and in the invasive carcinoma. The p16INK4a immunostaining showed diffuse and intense positivity throughout the dysplastic epithelium and in the areas of invasive carcinoma.

Table 1. The clinico-pathological features of the squamous cell carcinoma arising in epidermal cyst: review of the present study

Nr.	Age/sex	Clinical presentation	Treatment	Macroscopic features	Follow up
1	88/man	Right zigomatic area	Tumorectomy	Cystic mass of 7 mm. in maximum diameter	Free of disease 28 months after tumorectomy
2	96/man	Nodular lesion of the right helix	Tumorectomy	Cystic mass *tumour* of 1.6x1x1 cm	Free of disease 18 months after tumorectomy
3	67/man	Ulcerated nodular lesion of the right helix	Tumorectomy	Cystic mass of 8 mm. in maximum diameter	Free of disease 12 months after tumorectomy
4	86/man	Nodular lesion of the left helix	Tumorectomy	Cystic mass of 1.5 mm. in maximum diameter	Free of disease 8 months after tumorectomy
5	68/man	Cheek	Tumorectomy	Cystic mass of 1.6 mm. in maximum diameter	Free of disease 24 months after tumorectomy
6	61/man	Right ear	Tumorectomy	Cystic mass of 1.2 mm. in maximum diameter	Free of disease 24 months after tumorectomy
7	84/man	right forearm	Tumorectomy	Cystic mass of 1.5 mm. in maximum diameter	Free of disease 24 months after tumorectomy

Computed tomography with the administration of intravenous contrast material was performed for staging of malignancy and showed diffuse wall thickening of the anorectum and infiltration of anus levator's muscle *muscles'levator* (Figure 4, arrows). Endoscopic biopsies of the anal canal and rectum revealed squamous cell carcinoma with presence of HPV 16 (Figure 5). The patient has refused every treatment.

DISCUSSION

16 cases of SCC arising in EC have been reported to date (table I) (1-2-3-4-5-6-7-8-9-10-11-12-13-14). Lopez Rios et al (8) reviewed 27 cases reported in the English literature. These authors identified only 7 cases in which microscopic description and adequate figures corresponded to "SCC arising in a cutaneous epidermal cyst". On the other hand Miller's (3) and Yaffe's (4) cases had not complete histological illustrations. Some considerations can be

made about this small serie because it includes some curious cases. The 21-year-old woman reported by Morgan et al (11) is the youngest patient with cutaneous SCC described in the literature. The case reported by Debaize et al (12), with a size of 20 cm and a weight of 1.535 g, is the biggest one described in the literature. In conclusion a lesion may be diagnosed as "SCC arising in an EC" only with the support of an accurate histological documentation in order to exclude mimics (proliferating epidermoid cyst, proliferating trichilemmal cyst and pseudocarcinomatous hyperplasia in a ruptured cyst). HPV demonstration has to be negative in order to exclude a verrucous cyst. The main histological feature essential for diagnosis is the presence of a "continuum" between cystic wall and SCC *squamous cell carcinoma* proliferation. Appling this diagnostic criterion many reported cases shouldn't been classified in this group. Despite the low risk of malignant transformation, it is generally agreed that all suspected cutaneous cysts should be submitted for histological examination. In 1982 Meyer et al (1) described 5 cases of verrucous cysts (VCs), in which they detected HPV genomes by polymerase chain reaction (PCR), without specifying HPV type. The specific HPV type in VC was not been identified until 1992, when Matsukura et al (2) cloned HPV type from a cyst that showed non homology with other known prototypes of HPV (from HPV 1 through HPV 59), so that it was named HPV 60. In 1998, Egawa K et al (6) detected HPV 57 DNA by PCR and ISH in the plantar cyst of a 23-years old Japanese man. VCs most commonly arise in the palmoplantar regions (15-16-17), although similar lesions have been reported on the scalp (18), face (19-20), neck (20), trunk (18-20-21), arm (20-21) and leg (20). VCs have been described adjacent to warty lesions (22-23-24) in patients after organ transplantation. HPV infection is associated with a broad spectrum of human diseases, ranging from subclinical lesions to benign and malignant conditions (25-26). HPV 6 and 11 are usually associated with benign diseases (low risk HPV) (25-26). HPV 16 and 18 and, to some extent 33 and 31, are often associated with malignant diseases (high-risk HPV) (25-26). This is the first case report documenting the presence of HPV 16 in VC (22-27). Functionally high risk HPV types infection contributes to carcinogenesis and tumour progression predominantly through the action of two viral oncogenes, E6 and E7. The coordinated expression of E6 and E7 has been town to transform rodent cells and immortalize primary human keratinocytes (28-29). The E6 and E7 proteins of high-risk HPVs have been demonstrated to be able to associate with the products of p53 and retinoblastoma susceptibility (Rb) genes, respectively, and inactivate the functions of these tumour suppressor proteins (30-31). The E6 protein exerts rapid degradation of p53, in corporation with E6-associated protein (E6-AP), via ubiquitinmediated proteolysis pathway (32-33). The E7 protein mediates the release of the E2F transcription factor from pRb-E2F complex (34). Mutational analysis of HPV 16 E6 protein revealed that a certain level of the activity to degrade p53 is required for E6 to manifest its transforming function (35). The p53 mutations are the most frequent genetic abnormalities found in a wide variety of human malignant tumours (36). Once DNA damage occurs, p53 protein is induced and arrests cells in the G1 phase to enhance DNA repair (37), or triggers apoptosis following DNA damage (38). These functions of p53 protein are important to maintain the genomic integrity. Mutant p53 proteins are devoid of these functions, because they lose the ability of DNA contact or destabilize the structure of the core domain (29). In this way, once p53 is mutated, DNA damage is fixed and subsequent genetic rearrangement progress which may be putative mechanisms to initiate cancer. p16^{INK4a} is commonly expressed in cervical dysplasias and carcinomas associated with high risk HPV. Confirmation of high grade squamous intraepithelial abnormality is provided by the so-called "block-positivity", i.e.

immunoreactivity involving every cell in the complete, or almost complete, thickness of the squamous neoplastic epithelium (39). In our case $p16^{INK4a}$ immunostaining showed diffuse and intense positivity throughout the cystic epithelium and in the areas of invasive carcinoma confirming the presence of a high risk HPV in the cystic wall and in the invasive SCC *squamous carcinoma*. High risk HPV types may induce malignant transformation in other cutaneous lesions as viral acanthoma and papillomas of long duration (40). Approximately 72% of invasive anal cancer cases are *were* associated with HPV 16 and/or 18 infections (41). This estimate of 16 HPV and 18 prevalence is similar to the found in invasive cervical cancer cases (42). Anal cancer is a slowly progressing disease that begins as a superficial mass and may spread locally, involve regional lymph nodes or metastasize to distant organs (43). The pathogenesis of a simultaneous HPV infection of both anal canal and VC is unclear. The modality of VC infection by HPV is not known. Two hypotheses may exist: 1. the epidermis infected by HPV could have been implanted into the dermis; 2. HPV could initially have infected the upper part of eccrine duct, such as the acrosyringeal epithelium and then could have migrated into various parts of the dermal portions of the eccrine duct, where the virus-associated epidermoid cysts developed. The eccrine duct was not evident because of neoplastic destruction. A previous sexual contact could be responsible for anal infection by HPV 16, considering that carcinogenetic effect of infection may have a long latency period. Regarding our case of VC, the site, the malignant transformation, the finding of HPV 16 type and the extensive neoplastic involvement of adjacent organ may be considered features of an extraordinary rare case.

Table 2. Squamous cell carcinoma arising in cutaneous epidermal cysts: review of the literature

Authors	Age/Sex	Site	Duration of lesion	Size of cyst (cm)	Treatment	Outcome
Davidson et al. (1976)	52 M	L frontal region	2 months	NS	Excision	Free of disease
Bauer et al. (1980)	68 M	R retroauricular area	4 months	3	Excision + parotidectomy	Free of disease
Miller et al. (1981)	34 M	L retroauricular area	NS	8	Excision + RT 5,325 R	Free of disease after 25 years
Yaffe et al. (1982)	58 M	R ear	11 years	2.5	Excision	Free of disease
Arianayagam et al. (1987)	59 F	L tight	3 months	7	Excision + inguinal dissection	Lymph node metastasis; died after 6 months
Shah et al. (1989)	55 F	L gluteal region	6 months	10	Excision	NS
Davies et al. (1994)	32 M	L index finger	10 years	NS	Amputation + RT	Free of disease
López-Ríos et al. (1999)	66 M	L retroauricular area	2 months	1.5	Excision	Free of disease

Table 2. (Continued)

Authors	Age/Sex	Site	Duration of lesion	Size of cyst (cm)	Treatment	Outcome
Malone et al. (1999)	92 F	R forehead	NS	NS	Excision	No recurrence after 10 months
Wong et al. (2000)	57 NS	L buttock	20 years	6	Excision	Free of disease after 6 months
Morgan et al. (2001)	5 cases, 21-80 (mean age 56,7) 3 M, 2 F	Face, Neck, Trunk.	NS	NS	Excision	Free of disease (mean follow-up 2-6 years)
Debaize et al. (2002)	38 F	L buttock area	Since adolescence	20x15	Excision	Free of disease after 1 year
Cameron et al. (2003)	67 M	R temple	3 months	3	Excision	Free of disease after 6 months
Chiu et al. (2007)	74 M	Prossimal L thigh	40 years	15	Excision	Free of disease after 2 years

NS: not stated; RT: radiotherapy; L: left; R: right; M: male; F: female; SCC: squamous cell carcinoma.

REFERENCES

[1] Davidson T. M., Bone R. C., Kiessling P. J. Epidermoid carcinoma arising from within an epidermoid inclusion cyst. *Ann. Otol. Rhinol. Laryngol.* 1976 85,417-8.

[2] Bauer B. S., Lewis V. L. Carcinoma arising in sebaceous and epidermoid cysts. *Ann. Plast. Surg.* 1980 5 222-6 4.

[3] Miller J. M. Squamous cell carcinoma arising in an epidermal cyst. *Arch. Dermatol.* 1981 117,683.

[4] Yaffe H. S. Squamous cell carcinoma arising in an epidermal cyst. *Arch. Dermatol.* 1982 118,961.

[5] Arianayagam S., Jayalakshmi P. Malignant epidermal cyst: a case report. *Malaysian J. Pathol.* 1987 9,89-91.

[6] Shah L. K., Rane S. S., Holla V. V. A case of squamous cell carcinoma arising in an epidermal cyst. *Indian J. Pathol. Microbiol.* 1989 32, 138-140.

[7] Davies M. S., Nicholson A. G., Southern S., Moss A. H. L. Squamous cell carcinoma arising in a traumatically induced epidermal cyst. *Injury* 1994 25,116-7.

[8] López-Ríos F., Rodríguez-Peralto J. L., Castaño E., Benito A. Squamous cell carcinoma arising in a cutaneous epidermal cyst: case report and literature review. *Am. J. Dermatopathol.* 1999 21,174-7.

[9] Malone J. C., Sonnier G. B., Hughes A. P., Hood A. F. Poorly differentiated squamous cell carcinoma arising within an epidermoid cyst. *Int. J. Dermatol.* 1999 38,556-8.

[10] Wong T. H., Khoo A. K., Tan P. H., Ong B. H. Squamous cell carcinoma arising in a cutaneous epidermal cyst-a case report. *Ann. Acad. Med. Singapore*.2000 29,757-9.

[11] Morgan M. B., Stevens G. L., Somach S., Tannenbaum M. Carcinoma arising in epidermoid cyst: a case series and aetiological investigation of human papillomavirus. *Br. J. Dermatol.* 2001 145,505-6.

[12] Debaize S., Gebhart M., Fourrez T., Rahier I., Baillon J. M. Squamous cell carcinoma arising in a giant epidermal cyst: a case report. *Acta. Chir. Belg.* 2002 102,196-8.

[13] Cameron D. S., Hilsinger R. L. Jr. Squamous cell carcinoma in an epidermal inclusion cyst: case report. *Otolaryngol Head Neck Surg.* 2003 129,141-3.

[14] Chiu M. Y., Ho S. T. Squamous cell carcinoma arising from an epidermal cyst. *Hong Kong Med. J.* 2007 13,482-4.

[15] Egawa K., Inaba Y., Ono T., Arao T. 'Cystic papilloma' in humans? Demostration of humnan papillomavirus in plantar epidermoid cysts. *Arch. Dermatol.* 1990 126, 1599-603.

[16] Egawa K., Honda Y., Inaba. Y., Ono T., DeVilliers E.M. *et al.* Detection of human papillomaviruses and eccrine ducts in palmoplantar epidermoid cysts. *Br. J. Dermatol.* 1995 132,533-42.

[17] Rios-Buceta L. M., Fraga-Fernandez J., Femandez-Herrera J. Human *Hurman* papillomavirus in an epidermoid cyst of the sole in a non-Japanese patient. *J. Am. Acad. Dermatol.* 1992 27,364-6.

[18] Elston D. M., Parker L. U., Tuthill R P. J. Epidermoid cyst of the scalp containing human papillomavirus. *J. Cutan. Pathol.* 1993 20,184-6.

[19] Aloi F., Tomasini *Tornasini* C., Pippione M. HPV-related follicular cysts. *Am. J. Dermatopathol.* 1992 14,37-41.

[20] Soyer H. P., Schadendorf D., Cerroni L., Kerl H. Verrucous cysts: histopathologic characterization and molecular detection of human papillomavirus-specific DNA. *J. Cutan. Pathol.* 1993 20,411-7.

[21] Meyer L. M., Tyring S. K., Littie W. P. Verrucous cyst. *Arch. Dermatol.* 1991 127,1810-2.

[22] Egawa K., Kitasato H., Honda Y., Kawai S., Mizushima Y., Ono T. Human papillomavirus 57 identified in a plantar epidermoid cyst. *Br. J. Dermatol.* 1998 138,510-4.

[23] Jung K-D., Kim P-S., Lee J-H., Yang J-M., Lee E-S., Lee D-Y., Jang K-T., Kim D-S. Human papillomavirus-associated recurrent plantar epidermal cysts in a patient after organ transplantation. *J. Eur. Acad. Dermatol. Venereol.* 2009 23,837-9.

[24] Egawa K., Egawa N., Honda Y. Human papillomavirus-associated plantar epidermoid cyst related to epidermoid metaplasia of the eccrine duct epithelium: a combined histological, immunohistochemical, DNA-DNA in situ hybridization and three-dimensional reconstruction analysis. *Br. J. Dermatol.* 2005 152,961-967.

[25] McMurray H. R., Nguyen D., Westbrook T. F., McAnce D. l. Biology of human papillomaviruses. *Int. J. Exp. Pathol.* 2001 82,15-33

[26] Nebesio C. L., Mirowski G. W., Chuang T. Y. Human papillomavirus: clinical significance and malignant potential. *Int. J. Dermatol.* 2001 40,373-9.

[27] Kitasato H., Egawa K., Honda Y., Ono T., Mizushima Y., Kawai S. A putative human papillomavirus type 57 new subtype isolated from plantar epidermoid cysts without intracytoplasmic inclusion bodies. *J. Gen. Virol.* 1998 79,1977-81.

[28] Kanda T., Watanabe S., *and* Yoshiike K. Immortalization of primary rat cells by human papillomavirus type 16 subgenomic DNA fragment controlled by SV40 promoter. *Virology* 1988 165,321-5.

[29] Cho Y., Gorina S., Jeffrey P. D., *and* Pavletich N. P. Crystal structure of a p.53 tumor suppressor-DNA complex: understanding tumorigenic mutations. *Science* 1994 265, 346-55.

[30] Munger K., Werness B. A., Dyson N., Phelps W. C., Harlow E., *and* Howley P. M. Complex formation of human papillomavirus E7 proteins with theretinoblastoma tumor suppressor gene product. *EMBO J.* 1989 8, 4099-105.

[31] Werness B. A., Levine A. J., *and* Howley P. M. Association of human papillomavirus types 16 and 18 E6 proteins with p.53. *Science* 1990 248,76-9.

[32] Scheffner M., Werness B. A., Huibregtse J. M., Levine A. J. , *and* Howley P. M. The E6 oncoprotein encoded by human papillomavirus types 16 and 18 promotes the degradation of p.53. *Cell* 1990 *1993* 63, 1129-36.

[33] Huibregtse J. M., Scheffner M., *and* Howley P. M. Cloning and expression of the cDNA for E6-AP, a protein that mediates the interaction of the human papillomavirus E6 oncoprotein with p.53. *Mol. Cell Biol.* 1993 13,775-84.

[34] Nevins J. R. E2F: A link between the Rb tumor suppressor protein and viral oncoproteins. *Science* 1992 258, 424-9.

[35] Nakagawa S., Watanabe S., Yoshikawa H., Taketani Y., Yoshiike K. , *and* Kanda T. Mutational analysis of human papillomavirus type 16 E6 protein: transforming function for human cells and degradation of p.53 in vitro. *Virology* 1995 *1992*; 212, 535-42.

[36] Harris C. C. p53: At the crossroads of molecular carcinogenesis and risk assessment. *Science* 1993 262, 1980-1.

[37] Kuerbitz S. J., Plunkett B. S., Walsh W. V. , *and* Kastan M. B. Wild-type p53 *p.53* is a cell cycle checkpoint determinant following irradiation. *Proc. Natl. Acad. Sci.* US 1992 89, 7491-5.

[38] Lowe S. W., Schmitt E. M., Smith S. W., Osborne B. A. , *and* Jacks T. p53 *p.53* is required for radiation-induced apoptosis in mouse thymocytes. *Nature* 1993 362, 847-9.

[39] Mulvany N. J., Allen D. G., Wilson S. M. Diagnostic utility of p16[INK4a]: a reappraisal of its use in cervical biopsies. *Pathology.* 2008 40,335-44.

[40] Zur Hausen H. Papillomaviruses in human cancer. *Cancer.* 1987 59,1692-6.

[41] Austin, D. F.: Etiological clues from descriptive epidemiology: squamous carcinoma of the rectum or anus. *Natl. Cancer Inst. Monogr.* 1982 62, 89-90.

[42] Smith J. S., Lindsay L., Hoots B., Keys J., Franceschi S., Winer R., Clifford G.M. *et al.* Human papillomavirus type distribution in invasive cervical cancer and high-grade cervical lesions: a meta-analysis update. *Int. J. Cancer* 2007 121,621-32.

[43] Roach S. C., Hulse P. A., Moulding F. J., Wilson R., Carrington B.M. *et al* Magnetic resonance imaging of anal cancer. *Clin. Radiol.* 2005 60,1111-9.

INDEX

C

H

I

J

K

L

T